Football Fitness
and Injuries

LANCHESTER LIBRARY, Coventry University

Much Park Street   Coventry CVI 2HF   TEL. 0203 838292

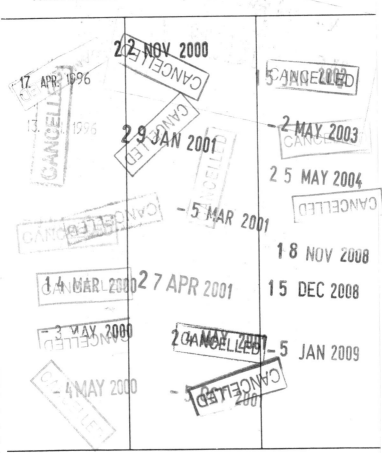

This book is due to be returned no later than the date stamped above.
Fines are charged on overdue books

Football Fitness and Injuries

*David Sutherland Muckle
and Harold Shepherdson*

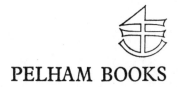

PELHAM BOOKS

First published in Great Britain by
PELHAM BOOKS LTD
52 Bedford Square
London WC1B 3EF
FEBRUARY 1975
SECOND IMPRESSION DECEMBER 1976

ISBN 0 7207 0801 X

Printed in Great Britain by
Hollen Street Press at Slough
and bound by Redwood Burn at Esher.

Contents

Illustrations

Illustrations

Acknowledgements

We would like to express our appreciation of all the kindness and help given by so many people, especially Margaret Stevenson M.A. who checked the manuscripts, Robert Emanuel (Department of Photography, Nuffield Orthopaedic Centre, Oxford) who produced the photographs, all who contributed to the 'Forewords' and criticised the manuscript and gave helpful suggestions, to the Staff of Oxford United who showed an unfailing interest and co-operation especially in the medical tests, to Harry and Cathy Burbidge who checked the proofs.

Dedication

To my wife Christine, and my daughters Carolyn and Deborah; and to my very good friends in Oxford and the North.

David.

To my wife Peggy, to Margaret and all my family.

Harold.

Forewords

1. By Sir Norman Chester C.B.E., M.A. (Oxon), M.A. (Admin) (Manc), Litt D., the author of the 'Chester Report' on professional soccer, of the 1966–68 Committee on Association Football. Nuffield College, Oxford.

Three quarter million play soccer each week in this country during the season. It is not a dangerous game but as each player strives hard, making great demands on his legs and body, strains and more serious injuries are bound to occur. In the case of the highly paid professional these can reduce his earnings and jeopardise his career. But even the most casual amateurs will suffer if injuries received during a match are not treated quickly and expertly. Here is a book specially designed to help every club and player. Harold Shepherdson is known throughout the professional game as a first class trainer. Mr David Muckle has specialised in accidents and injuries. Both can draw on a wide practical experience of soccer injuries. Together they make a powerful team. Their book should be widely welcomed.

Norman Chester.

2. By John Cockin, M.A., M.B., Ch.B., F.R.C.S., F.R.C.S.E., Consultant Orthopaedic and Accident Surgeon, Consultant in Charge of the Accident Service, Radcliffe Infirmary, Oxford, Research Fellow, Hertford College, Oxford.

The treatment of any injury begins at the time of the injury itself and frequently the eventual outcome and recovery can be determined by the prompt and speedy attention which is given on the spot. It is equally true, of course, that many accidents can – and should – be prevented. In this book the adoption of correct training methods should do much not only to prevent injuries but also to provide the sportsman with a degree of fitness so that he is able to overcome any disability at the earliest possible moment. The correct care of football injuries and of their immediate treatment is of prime importance. In the combination of David Muckle and Harold Shepherdson this book should provide a significant contribution not only to the prevention of injuries but also to the rapid recovery from an injury by ensuring that the initial treatment and after-care is correctly and efficiently applied.

John Cockin.

3. By Gordon Banks, O.B.E., former England Goalkeeper.

As England's team trainer through four World Cup competitions, Harold Shepherdson has had millions of pounds worth of Soccer talent pass through his hands – and I mean that literally. For as well as putting players through their paces on the training pitch, he has handled many of the injuries which beset any team from time to time.

As an England player who took part in the 1966 World Cup tournament, and who went with England to Mexico in 1970, I can vouch for Harold's skill and knowledge, for his ability to make training sessions lively and enjoyable, and to get footballers back into action in the swiftest possible time. 'Shep', as we have affectionately called him, knows his job right the way through. Over the years we have come to appreciate that physical and mental well-being are important – vital in fact – for professional footballers, and that effective treatments for injuries is a basic requisite for fielding a team of players at their peak. In this book Harold Shepherdson has called on his detailed knowledge, in combination with the orthopaedic and sports injury expertise of Mr David S. Muckle, who has had a close association with many first class and international players in football, cricket, rugger and athletics. I am delighted to pay my own testimony to this work, an I am sure that this book will be of tremendous benefit to everyone who reads it.

Gordon Banks.

4. *By Frank O'Gorman, M.R.C.P., F.R.C.S., F.R.C.O.G., Professor Associate in Surgery, University of Sheffield, Director, Sheffield United F.C., Hon. Physician, The Football Association.*

The authors of this book make an ideal combination. Both are athletes, one an ex-amateur and the other an ex-professional footballer, one an orthopaedic surgeon, and the other a coach and physiotherapist with a wide experience of the treatment of soccer injuries at club and international levels.

They have demonstrated their ability to express their ideas in simple and lucid fashion, and in that respect they differ from many so-called experts. They have clearly explained basic principles in relation to fitness and injury, and throughout the book they have stressed the importance of common sense in diagnosis and treatment.

All will agree that the right time to treat an injury is immediately after it has occurred. In this respect our professional clubs, with doctor and physiotherapist on the spot, not to mention the availability of modern equipment, have few problems. Those of us, however, who conduct sports injury clinics for amateur athletes will welcome the publication of this book because it will help the scores of ordinary trainers and coaches to deal urgently and properly with the injuries of the many thousands of day to day sportsmen who derive such enjoyment from their week-end games, but who can suffer much disability and loss of work from initially poor and not infrequently over-enthusiastic treatment.

It is for these reasons – better primary therapy and earlier return to work and sports activity – that I hope this book will become part of the equipment of most, if not all, clubs up and down the country. The authors have rendered a considerable service to sportsmen by writing it, and I personally hope that it achieves the success it deserves.

Frank O'Gorman.

5. By Emlyn Hughes, Liverpool and England.

This book explains the many problems relating to fitness and injury in football. Harold Shepherdson has had a vast experience as England's trainer for the past seventeen years and in this book in collaboration with David Muckle F.R.C.S. they have made their practical knowledge available as a guide to the many people who are connected with football at all levels.

Emlyn Hughes.

Introduction

No one can doubt that the standard of medical care given to sportsmen has improved during recent years, mainly due to the awakening of interest in 'Sports Medicine' by doctors and physiotherapists. There have also been vigorous efforts by the Football Association to encourage trainers to attend official courses on therapy and management. However, many small clubs still require the earnest endeavours of the amateur trainer or therapist who may find attendance at such courses difficult because of social or occupational commitments. Thus thousands of teams (school, college, works, club, village and town) continue to rely upon good fortune, outdated manuals and the empiricism of the bucket and sponge.

There is also no doubt that the best time to treat injuries is when they happen, but with what? and how? ... has the player suffered a fracture? ... is an X-ray needed? ... should heat be given? These are the simple questions which this book hopes to answer in a straightforward and lucid manner. The data is intended as a guide to some, and a reminder to others, and we hope it will provoke further reading and thought.

Good luck in your football.

D.S.M.,　　　　　　H.S.,
Woodstock,　　　　Middlesbrough,
OXON.　　　　　　 Teesside.

SPECIAL NOTE

Many of the treatments for injuries described in this book are strictly surgical/medical, and should only be carried out by surgeons or doctors, or under their supervision. Where first aid to the injured is concerned, the person giving such aid should follow the first precepts of first aid in moving the casualty as little as possible (or not at all where a spinal injury is likely), keeping him warm, etc., and enlisting medical assistance as soon as possible.

Chapter One

Injuries in Sport

The football trainer has a key role in the success of any club. He is the pivot in the defence against injuries. The first team coaching and selection absorbs much of the manager's attention. But no matter how well that team plays, it has a short life without adequate backing, especially the medical arrangements. How often the cry: 'We were going great guns in the League until injury struck.' What a sad spectacle it is to see potential match winners sitting on the bench, while their colleagues blunder on, bereft of inspiration.

The ideal situation consists of club doctor, specialist (usually orthopaedic), physiotherapist and coach working in close harmony. However, this ideal is rarely achieved, unless one considers the major professional teams. Thousands upon thousands of sportsmen rely upon the helpful advice and professional encouragement of the trainer. The players not only look to him for help with injuries but for intimate discussions on tricky personal problems. In his rôle as the father-figure the trainer must have a grasp of the principles of treatment, which in turn demands an understanding of anatomy and practical physiotherapy.

Bearing in mind all the ramifications of sports injuries, a motto for any up-and-coming young trainer should be: *Always adopt a positive approach to fitness, and to the treatment of ill-health.*

Let me give an example: a few years ago I can remember on two separate occasions star professional players being out of action due to ingrowing toe nails – not for days, but for months! In each case the diligence of the trainer could have prevented the condition by paying attention to footwear, foot hygiene and early treatment. Instead the club paid the penalty for neglect, and one of the players was lucky not to loose the tip of his toe due to an infection of the bone.

Luckily serious football injuries are uncommon, and as assessed by every 100 participants soccer causes fewer injuries than skiing and rugger. Many of my rugger friends argue at length about which is the most dangerous sport. Certainly my own casualty experiences indicate rugger and skiing, although some series (concerned with mortality rates) lay great stress on the dangers of swimming and bowls! However, the results of a recent survey are as follows:

Sports injury rate per hundred partaking:

Rugger	5%
Skiing	5%
Gymnastics	3%
Soccer	3%
Hockey	2.5%
Judo	2.1%
Boxing	1.7%
Basketball	1.7%

A review of the injury list at Oxford United in the 1972–73 and 1973–74 seasons showed that out of a playing staff of 22 professionals on average two players (less than 10 per cent) attended for minor medical matters weekly (i.e. grazes, sprains, small haematomas etc.) although minor infections (colds, influenza etc.) accounted for a further 1 per cent.

Although a certain number of injuries has to be expected, the quantity can be controlled by correct training techniques: a warm-up period, a positive approach to balanced nutrition, good personal hygiene (including teeth), a sound knowledge of each player's weakness and phobias, and immediate post-injury care. In fact, good common sense!

The injury rate of a typical football club with a staff of thirty is shown below (as published in a recent book on football management*):

Fractures	3	Tibia and fibula (simple and compound),
		Nose.
Joint Injuries	52	Mainly Knee Injuries (18), ankle (33), etc.
Muscle and Tendon Injuries	71	Mainly Quadriceps (20), hamstrings (13), groin (12), etc.
Upper Limb Injuries	3	Shoulder sprain (1), clavicular sprain (2).
Back Injuries	12	
Head Injuries	2	
Medical Conditions	22	
Miscellaneous	6	Wounds and abrasions, etc.
Total:	171	

The Football Managers – Pawson T., Eyre Methuen, London, 1973.

The following is a detailed examination of the injuries which caused players to miss matches at Oxford United in 1972–73:

Effusion/bleeding knee	3
Minor head injury	1
Shoulder sprain	1
Groin strain	1
Leg infection	2
Dislocated fibula	1
Fractured ankle	1 (player on loan to Plymouth Argyle)
In 60 matches:	10

Visiting players sustained: a fractured orbital bone, a minor head injury, a scalp laceration and a twisted ankle. One Oxford Reserve player fell off his bike and fractured his nose, another slipped against a training bench and twisted his knee. In all the injury rate was less than 1.5 per cent.

The dislocation of the fibula at the knee was an exceedingly uncommon injury caused by an awkward fall;* while the minor head injury was produced by heading a cross-ball and was associated with twenty minutes of confusion. The two infections of the shin occurred despite immediate cleansing with a mild antiseptic and the administration of oral antibiotics. Both infections required a plaster cast to the lower limb for five days. Incidently, these were the only occasions when a plaster cast was used as a primary procedure, and more will be stated on this subject later (Chapter 9). Three players were rested for over-use injuries at the shoulder and groin. A correct warming-up period ensured that no player developed a florid groin strain or other chronic injury.

*Reference: *British Journal of Sports Medicine*, page 365, 1973.

In a report from Arsenal* seven out of 53 players were attending for treatment at any one time, although most injuries were of a minor nature. The report emphasises the importance of the correct psychological approach in treating professional footballers. The injured man must feel he is still part of the team, even though he is doing special exercises. The psychological factor is nowhere better illustrated than in the treatment of an Arsenal player who received a compound fracture of the tibia and fibula.

'When I came off the field I thought I was finished,' he said. The shadows of Derek Dooley, the Sheffield Wednesday centre-forward who lost his leg with gas gangrene, and of Dave Mackay, the Tottenham wing-half, who lost a year of his career after breaking his leg, hang over many footballers.

Within three hours of the Arsenal player's injury, the fracture was plated in an operating theatre, using the technique of pressure plating, which obviates the need for plaster of Paris afterwards. Within two weeks, the player was attending the ground during training sessions, joining in body exercises, and he still felt part of the team. He watched all the games for the rest of the season, and was back in the first team in nine months.

In a series studied, top-class amateur players in the Northern League had an injury rate between 3.5 and 3.9 per cent, but this figure included many trivial injuries (grazes, cut eyes, minor haematomas etc.). Serious injuries accounted for less than 1 per cent, although there were more fractures (ankle, shin and clavicle) among these amateur players than is experienced with professional players. However, a report from Leeds has tended to find the reverse. One impression was that the fatigue found in amateur players during the last half an hour of a match tended to produce more pulled muscles and chronic ligament strains.

Thus if this introductory chapter has served its purpose it will have indicated the relatively low injury rate amongst soccer players, with the majority requiring brief medical attention

World Medicine, p. 17, 1:67.

and remedial therapy. However, the summation of repeated minor injuries can lead to the development of chronic injuries necessitating the abandonment of a sporting career in later years.

Each injury needs prompt attention to avoid further complications.

Chapter Two

What to do – and What Not to Do

Man has an inherent instinct to fuss the injured. This is easily witnessed at any minor domestic or road traffic accident, and often the attempted cure (born of ignorance) becomes far more dangerous than the injury. To rationalise treatment one must understand the negatives as well as the positives, and apply the first aid in a cool and collected manner. To overcome the primitive urge of fear and apprehension, often manifest in the therapist as well as the injured, the trainer needs knowledge and self-restraint. Knowledge is required to decide on the most beneficial course of treatment; restraint is needed to realise when a line has to be drawn between treatment and meddling.

In the case of a serious injury, check that:
If the player is not breathing normally, clear airway by placing the head to one side and downwards, or by elevating the tip of the jaw by pressing the chin firmly upwards (player lying on his back or side). If breathing stops, commence artificial respiration (figure 1).
Assess the level of consciousness, if unconscious place in the recovery position (figure 2).
Check for serious bleeding and control it with a pressure dressing.
Do not move the player unnecessarily to undress the injured area, cut off all clothes if need be.

If it is necessary to turn an injured player into the recovery position, you should:

1. Kneel beside him and place both his arms close to his body.
2. Turn the player gently on to his side (grasping the clothes at shoulder and hip).
3. Draw the upper arm towards the face so that it makes a right angle with the body.
4. Draw up the upper leg until the thigh makes a right angle with the body and bend the knee.
5. Extend the underneath arm behind the back.
6. Bend the undermost knee slightly.

The player is now in a stable position with the head to one side, the chances of any vomit or blood being inhaled are eliminated.

MOUTH TO MOUTH RESPIRATION AND EXTERNAL CARDIAC
MASSAGE

Firstly, feel for a pulse at the wrist or neck.

Then, if no pulse or heart beat is felt, commence mouth to mouth respiration and cardiac massage.

Mouth to mouth respiration. Clear the mouth of debris, lie the player on his back, extend the neck to open the airway and pinch the player's nose (to stop air coming down), take a deep breath and blow into the player's mouth until the chest rises. Take mouth away and air will rush out of his lungs. Repeat every six seconds.

External Cardiac Massage. Kneel beside the player, extend your elbows and cross both hands, placing the crossed palms on the lower part of the sternum (central breastbone). Press gently but firmly backwards depressing the chest wall for 1 in. then release. A pulse beat should be felt at the wrist, neck or groin with each massage. Repeat at the rate of sixty per minute (every second). After every fourth beat, allow the person doing mouth to mouth respiration to inflate the lungs.

Always place the player on a hard surface for external cardiac massage, use the floor, pitch or a wooden board, not a soft bed or blankets (since these materials will absorb the firm pressure).

External cardiac massage is tiring and persons should alternate every five minutes until the doctor arrives.

The first and most obvious place to begin is the field of play. The circumstances are common enough, namely the player lies crouching and clutching his shin after a heavy tackle with a distinct look of anguish on his countenance, the manager yells a multitude of directions from the line, the trainer looks in puzzlement at the swelling limb, the referee consults his watch with a grave and solemn air, and the players mill round in idle knots.

The first positive action the trainer has to take is to decide whether the bone is broken or dislocated; *the first thing he must not do is to attempt a reduction of the injured part.*

Let us suppose, for example, that the player complains of a severe shoulder pain after an awkward fall, and that the normal smooth outline of the shoulder is lost, with limited movements and muscle spasm. A diagnosis of a dislocated shoulder is made – it may even have been recurrent, the trainer having seen it on the same player many times before. Thus he feels justified in attempting a reduction to ease suffering and prevent further soft tissue damage. Alas, what is not realised is that in this case the humerus is broken at its neck as well as dislocated, and attempted reduction causes more pain and aggravates the injury.

It is a simple rule that if a deformity is present then the bone must be broken or dislocated.

But there are other features of bone injury, and these are listed below. All trainers must be able to recognise a fracture or dislocation, and they are not always as painful as one would imagine. I recall one player training and playing for three weeks with a fractured shaft of fibula until he was referred to the X-ray department.

(a) Fractures and Dislocations

The Classical signs of a fracture are:

deformity, only absent with a crack fracture;

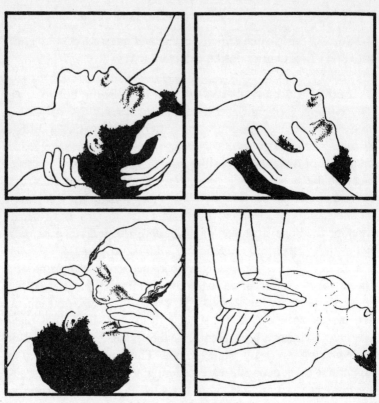

1. Mouth to mouth respiration.

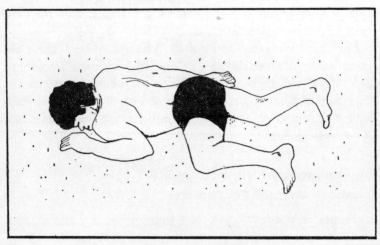

2. The recovery position.

pain, usually sharp and severe, with localisation to the bone;
abnormal mobility of the bone;
crepitus or grating of the bone ends;
loss of function, unlike sprains or bruises of soft tissues, a fracture means that the player cannot exert force against resistance;
bone tenderness, which means tenderness accurately localised to the surface of the bone and not to the soft tissues above. This is a sure sign of fracture.

The classical signs of a dislocation are:

pain, which is usually severe or sickly in nature, and occurs near a joint;

loss of movement, at the joint due to pain, and muscle spasm;
deformity, due to separation of the joint surfaces.

On very rare occasions the fracture or dislocation causes direct pressure on the blood vessels supplying the limb. Such embarrassment of the circulation is recognised by:

no pulse, below the injured area;

pallor, mottling or blueness (cyanosis) of the skin;

reduced warmth and tingling of the nerves in the limb.

If the trainer suspects complications such as those mentioned above, medical advice should be sought urgently.

Fractures can be open or closed, and the latter are called simple fractures. However, it is the open or compound fractures which are liable to infections because the skin over the injured area is broken and bacteria can readily invade the damaged tissues. Later the invading germs produce abscess formation, cellulitis and osteomyelitis (or infected bones). These are serious complications and are only avoided by meticulous medical care. As a first aid measure the damaged area is covered with a sterile dressing and splinted to prevent further damage.

Always apply splints to the limbs in a careful manner, do

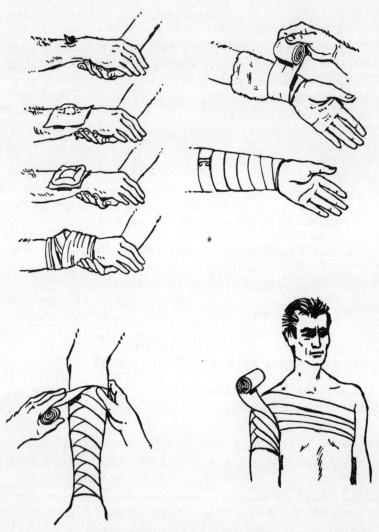

3. Methods of applying a sterile dressing.

not wobble the injured parts. Remember the maxim: 'Splint them where they lie.'

Dressings and bandages
A *dressing* is a protective covering applied to a wound to:
prevent infection;
control bleeding;
absorb discharge;
avoid further injury.

The dressing must be germ-free (sterile) if possible. It should also have a high degree of porosity to allow the evaporation of sweat and secretions so that the injured area does not become moist and liable to infection.

A mesh dressing will promote blood clotting.

A non-adhesive dressing, on removal, will not tear or damage the newly grown tissues.　•

A bandage is used to:
maintain direct pressure over a dressing to control bleeding,
retain dressings and splints in position;
prevent or reduce swelling;
provide support for a limb or joint;
restrict movement;
assist in moving casualties.

Unless bandages are applied firmly they are useless, dressings and splints will slip, and bleeding may be made worse. When too tightly applied bandages will cut off the circulation to the limb or area involved and a bluish colour will be seen in the skin. This bluish tinge is most easily seen in the finger or toe nail beds. Bandages are made from flannel, calico, elastic net or special paper. However, they can be improvised from stockings, ties, scarves, belts etc.

Splints
If splints are required, they should be:

rigid;

long enough to immobilise the joint above and below the fracture;
well padded and wide enough to fit comfortably to the limb;
applied over clothing.

In emergencies, a splint may be improvised from a walking stick, piece of wood, broom handle, folded cardboard, etc.

Splints require to be bandaged firmly on to the injured limb, but not so tightly as to interfere with the circulation or to cause pain. Separate skin surfaces (e.g. between legs) with soft pad-

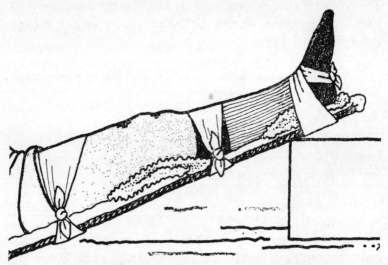

4. Splinting to immobilise above and below fracture.

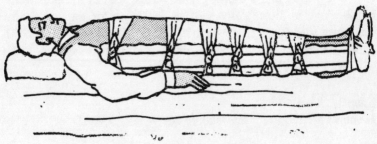

5. Splinting to immobilise the lower body.

ding before bandaging or splinting together. This action prevents discomfort and chafing.

Always slide the splint gently under the injured area, and move the limb as little as possible during application. Tie the knots over the splint or on the uninjured side. If both lower limbs are injured, tie the knots in front between them.

To pass bandages beneath the player use the natural hollows of the body, e.g. neck, loins, knees.

The canvas bed of a stretcher should be stiffened by placing short boards across it. If a blanket has to be placed under the player for warmth or lifting, roll the blanket or rug lengthwise for half its width and place the roll in line and against the casualty. Gently turn the player towards one side and push the rolled blanket under the back. The player is then rolled gently on to his opposite side and the blanket unrolled. The player is gently turned on to his back.

(b) Haemorrhage

Occasionally bleeding, which may be profuse, occurs from torn blood vessels, either with or without a fracture or dislocation. Now, cases are well documented when a limb has been completely severed in the course of battle or road accident and only a trivial amount of blood has been spilt. Indeed the surgeons of the fifteenth century relied upon swift severance of a limb (and an application of boiling tar, as a safeguard) during their amputations. The reason for the lack of blood loss is due to the fact that if a blood vessel is divided cleanly, it will contract due to spasm and cut off the haemorrhage. However, the incomplete or jagged tear will prevent contraction and the haemorrhage will continue unabated. What can the trainer do? Look for pressure points? ... possible, but inadequate except in the most extreme bleeding. Apply a tourniquet? ... often quite useless, because if too tightly tied the underlying vessels and nerves are strangled, and if too slackly applied then bleeding is encouraged.

The answer is to apply a pressure dressing. This means that the bleeding area is covered with a thick layer of dressings, cot-

B

ton wool and a fairly tight crêpe (elastic) bandage. This firm dressing, coupled with splinting of the limb, will control haemorrhage.

I know that many first-aiders will throw up their hands in horror at the apparent denigration of the time-honoured tourniquet. Although it may be argued that this device is useful in a limb with multiple bleeding areas, I have never known haemorrhage not be controlled by a firm pressure dressing, and this experience includes many severe multiple injuries.

Thus all trainers must be familiar with the application of pressure dressings. Don't rely on tourniquets or pressure points.

(c) Head Injuries

The brain is a semi-fluid substance, so any blow on the skull or face (including the chin) will impart momentum to the brain substance and it will wobble inside the skull. The magnitude of the blow determines the amount of brain deformation and the extent of head injury and possible unconsciousness.

When a player is *knocked out,* he may have:

a fractured skull;

bleeding from the veins or arteries within the skull; or

bruising to the brain substance.

One thing is certain, the player has suffered from some degree of temporary nerve damage – or he would not have been knocked out!

It should be a golden rule that all footballers rendered unconscious should leave the field, and not be allowed to return. To resume playing, which can increase the blood flow at least ten-fold through the tissues, will make any bleeding within the skull much worse.

It is quite common that once a player comes round from being knocked out, he appears to act quite normally – the so-called lucid period. This clear interval is then followed by a period of headache, confusion, nausea, vomiting, and eventual loss of consciousness. Blows on the temporal region (just above

34

the ear) are the worst offenders in this respect, so always beware of a confused player with a bruise on the temporal area,
he might be suffering from an intracranial bleed.

The correct treatment for a minor head injury is:

escort the player from the field once he has regained consciousness – using a stretcher is preferable to walking him across the
pitch;

keep him rested, and covered with a blanket until he reaches
hospital;

never give a drink to an injured player;

examine the neck to make sure he has not damaged his spine.

Many hospitals adopt the policy of keeping the once-
unconscious player in the wards for 24-hour observation, even
if the skull X-ray is negative for a fracture. This policy means
that should any deterioration in condition occur, then immediate
facilities for operation are on hand.

Often players seem to recover quickly from a minor head
injury, but the continuation of a confused state can be recognised
by their stereotyped behaviour (rather like a drunken man)
especially when it comes to asking the same question over and
over again e.g. 'What's the score' at intervals of every minute
or so. I recall one such incident in a match against Queens Park
Rangers when an apparently straightforward heading of the ball
caused a temporary loss of consciousness in a midfield player.
Luckily the trainer, Ken Fish, fully conversant with the facts
of minor head injuries, insisted on the immediate removal of the
player from the pitch. For the subsequent 20 minutes in the
dressing room the player was disorientated, asking 'What
time's the kick off?' although to every other intent and purpose
he seemed to behave rationally. The press photograph showed
the player leaving the field with what they captioned as a 'deep
interest in the fate of his colleagues', although in fact he was
completely unaware of his whereabouts.

In another match – an amateur cup quarter final – a player
received a blow to the head, and after being well and truly
drenched by spongefuls of cold water, was thrust back into the

game with apparent success. Unfortunately at half-time the player refused to leave field and continued an imaginary game on his own, until he was persuaded to come off by the match officials. Later hospital tests showed a depressed fracture of the skull which required an immediate operation.

Thus a head injury is more than a temporary lull in play, it could be a life-threatening accident. Do *not* allow players to return to the game after head injuries.

(d) Spinal Injuries

Occasionally an injured spine (especially the neck or cervical spine) may coexist with a head injury. This is because the neck is bent acutely forwards or backwards as the head strikes either a post, a player or the ground. Under these circumstances the neck may fracture (usually a crush fracture of the vertebral body) or dislocate. Although this is a very rare injury in footballers, being much more common in jockeys and huntsmen, I have observed it on isolated occasions, once noting this injury in a dental student who had walked around the Medical School continuing his duties and studies for a week until the unremitting neckache forced him to visit the Casualty Department. Goalkeepers can injure their necks as they dive over the ball at the feet on an on-rushing forward or collide with the goal post. The classic, and oft-quoted, case is that of the former Manchester City goalkeeper, Bert Trautmann, who played through the 1956 Cup Final against Birmingham City with a broken neck; later being voted Player of the Year.

Damage to the spine is denoted by:
severe pain in the back or neck, radiating to the arms, legs or trunk;

an inability to move the spine, arms or legs;

altered sensation, numbness or tingling in the arms or legs.

In all cases of spinal injury, the less the patient is moved around the better the prognosis. Handle the injured with care, and call for urgent medical advice with the player unmoved (i.e. still lying on the pitch). Forget about the match for a few moments! Do not transport the player unless he is conscious, a firm stretcher or wooden board (or door) available, and medical care is at hand. Do not roll the player from side to side; support the neck with the hands or small sandbags, and keep the head to one side if the player is vomiting.

One sees amazing things in football. I remember a First Division goalkeeper, having just completed a swallow-dive on to the nape of his neck, being hauled to his feet, rubbed with a sponge, cursorily examined, and thrown back into the arena. The next time he made contact with the ball he collapsed, although luckily a later X-ray did not show a fracture.

The rule is: *Never take chances with the spinal cord, all players with severe neck pain must come off for an X-ray.*

(e) No Drinks

This rather incongruous heading has nothing to do with the night before the match, nor does it relate to the frequent impecunious state some of my colleagues develop when adjacent to the club bar! It refers to that pernicious practice which I have observed in many clubs, including some in the First Division proud of their glorious past, of offering mouthfuls of cold water (or fruit juice, or tea) to an injured player before the extent of his injury is known. It is a golden rule in medical circles, hallowed by all anaesthetists, that an anaesthetic will *not* be given until a period of four hours has elapsed since the last drink or food. Even a sip of fluid is not allowed!

The unwary trainer who gives an injured player a drink may:

pour it directly into the larynx (windpipe) if the player is confused or semi-conscious;

cause retching, vomiting and then inhalation or regurgitation of stomach contents;

delay a life-saving or necessary anaesthetic for four hours.

Never give a drink or food to an injured player until after he has been examined by a doctor. Remember this fact, and the whole chapter has been worthwhile!

Once the player has left the field and the excited manager informed and sedated to control his natural tendency to rush his 'star' back to the foray (this is not an exaggeration, for I recall one manager refusing to allow his injured player to leave the field) there are several more 'Don'ts' to observe:

do not stick dirty creams or pastes on cuts and abrasions; you will be amazed at how many bacteria and fungi can be grown from old jars which have collected the dressing room dust of ages. A simple cleansing of the wound with mild liquid antiseptic will suffice, followed by a sterile dressing.

do not decide to have another look if a wound is covered on transit to a medical centre or hospital.

do not say to the player: "Just stand on that leg again, son, and jog up and down!' You cannot run off injuries, no more than you can run a faulty car-engine, without inflicting further damage. (Horrific tales of broken bones being driven through the skin by 'running-off' injuries are not unknown).

(f) Recent Injuries

The correct procedure with recent injuries is to immobilise the injured limb in crêpe and wool or plaster for at least twenty-four hours, then gentle body exercises and static exercises can begin.

Like moths drawn to a flame, the jet-set soccer player is attracted to discos and parties. As much as it goes against the grain, the injured player must realise that the damaged area needs rest and will not suffer the ingratitudes of a Saturday night out. The limb must be elevated in a sling or on a stool for long periods to reduce the swelling, and eventually the period of incapacity will be shortened. Undue activity at this early stage – and this includes standing – can only increase the oedema and make matters worse.

Finally there is the period of non-therapy to the injured part. Nature will heal in its own time, and, as yet, there is no magic pill which will heal fractures or soft-tissues faster than nature ordains. Rest aids recovery, while vigorous massage and undue heat (either infra-red or ultrasound) prolongs incapacity if given too early. I am still puzzled when I visit many minor clubs to see recently injured players having immediate heat-therapy, with legs that look like grilled kippers from the repeated exposure to heat over the season. If one wishes to increase the blood supply to the injured area and the amount of bleeding, then heat away!

As a general rule: *Sack anyone who heats an injured area within forty-eight hours, or while swelling is increasing.* He is not only increasing the period of incapacity and giving the opposition points, he is encouraging more swelling and fibrosis. It is best to remember that recent muscle injuries cannot be:

run off;
heated away;
massaged away;
stretched, pulled or manipulated away;
electrically stimulated away; or
injected away.

There is an art in doing nothing. The natural healing tendencies of the body can be advantageously employed, and providing that remedial and medical therapy is slowly, exactly, and gently incorporated into this quiescent phase of tissue healing, then the final result will be favourable.

In a nutshell: 'They also serve who only watch and wait.'

Chapter Three

Soft Tissue Injuries – Acute

Soft tissue injuries include damage to muscles, tendons, ligaments, capsules, fascia and skin. They may occur on their own or with a fracture or dislocation. When a bone is broken the principal interest of the doctor or physiotherapist is often directed away from the coincidental soft tissue trauma, but the latter injury may turn out to be the most important, and incapacitating, in the long run. I have seen promising young athletes and footballers recover from broken bones, so that on the final X-ray the fracture could not be detected. However, the soft tissue scarring and muscle atrophy had been such that a permanent fall off in performance ended their career.

In any fracture or dislocation the forces needed to break the bone or disrupt the joint must always injure the ensheathing soft tissues.

When treating a fracture or dislocation regard must be given to the associated soft tissue damage, and any therapy designed to promote the maximum recovery in all tissues.

X-rays at Oxford support the above dictum, for they show a soundly united tibia following a crack fracture, and yet one year later the young professional player was unable to play football at higher levels because of the resulting scar tissue in the muscles and fascia around the fracture. His mobility, jumping and sprinting powers were impaired and he eventually lowered his grade of football to semi-professional levels. Thus despite excellence on X-rays, the limiting factor was soft tissue damage.

Over 90 per cent of all the trainers' activities will concern soft tissues, and an understanding of their basic components is necessary. The main component of tendons, ligaments, fascia and bones is a fibre known as collagen, which gives strength to these structures, while allowing a certain degree of stretching. However, once soft tissues have been unduly stretched then another fibre with elastic properties, lying amongst the collagen fibres, produces recoil so that the part regains its original size. This fibre is known as elastin. The amount of both fibrous tissues varies from area to area, being dense in tendons and ligaments, but widely spread in the layers under the skin. The amount of fibrous tissue distributed amongst the muscle fibres also varies, and in animals gives rise to the variation in tenderness which characterises a rump or fillet steak. However, after a sudden stretching force has overtaxed the resources of these fibres, some may snap, producing what we recognise as a sprain, strain or tendon rupture.

It is also obvious that when one structure around a joint is

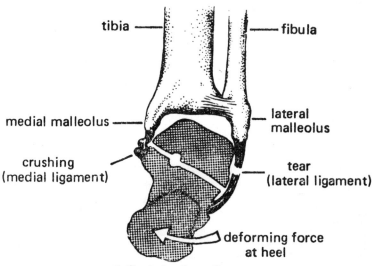

6. Crushed and torn ligaments.

stretched, another may be squashed, as the accompanying drawing shows.

However, the torn fibres must be repaired, and this is where complicating factors begin to operate. Cells produce new collagen and elastic fibres in abundance, which eventually shows as scar tissue and adhesions. These unwanted tissues bind down tendons, ligaments, muscles, blood vessels and nerves, interfering with the normal smooth movement of the limb, and producing tender, painful areas. *The secret of good soft tissue repair is to obtain a strong yet pliant scar.*

The strength of the scar is obtained by strict rest and the pliancy by graduated exercises. Since it takes several weeks for collagen fibres to be laid down, a tear in a joint capsule, ligament or tendon will not be strong enough for sporting use for at least three weeks. If the injured part is stressed before the collagen has had time to be correctly orientated then the newly arranged fibres are retorn, more collagen is laid down, the scar becomes denser and the playing ability grinds to a halt.

Never rush an athlete back to full activity before he is competent in remedial exercises or training; if he breaks down then the injury will be aggravated and confidence lost.

Muscle Injuries

Injuries to muscle are caused by *direct* blows (such as a kick to the thigh) or *indirect* forces (such as a pulled groin muscle). There is an essential difference between the two types of injury. Direct injuries are associated with swelling (muscle haematoma) and pain relative to the degree of injury observed, but indirect injuries are found without an easily discernible swelling, bleeding or lump while the pain is out of all proportion to the signs. No one can doubt the terrific pain of a pulled hamstring, yet little may be obvious on clinical examination. This means that the trainer or doctor has to rely upon the subjective impressions of the player to ascertain the value of his treatment. Players suffering from a lack of form often resort to pulled or indirect injuries as an excuse, and their treatment relies on psychology as well as remedial therapy.

When a muscle is damaged it bleeds. This may seem an obvious and pedantic remark, but it is the restriction of bleeding which is a prerequisite in muscle treatment. A second and equally important point is to remember that muscle fibres have little or no power of regeneration. Thus a damaged area in muscle is replaced by scar tissue, and many soccer players have hard nodules in the thigh and calf muscles due to previous damage. If the scar tissue becomes marked then muscle power becomes reduced, leading to poor running, turning and jumping.

It is essential to limit the amount of damage to muscle tissue, since the injured fibres can never recover.

How does one treat muscle injuries? During the acute stage the injured limb is rested in a plaster or crêpe and wool support, and the amount of swelling should be controlled by the application of cold to the injured area; ice cubes in a rubber bottle (which can be moulded around the part) is an excellent way. Ice therapy is given for 30–60 minutes. A cautionary note – never apply ice directly to the skin or the tissues will freeze, leading to small ulcers. The swelling can also be reduced by elevating

INTERMUSCULAR

INTRAMUSCULAR

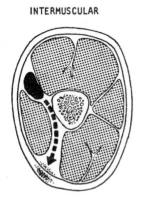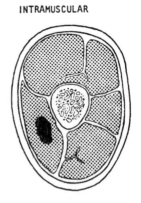

7. Muscle haematoma – cross-section through thigh.

43

the arm in a sling or the leg on a bench. This therapy is called I.C.E. – Ice, Compression and Elevation.

Muscle injuries can be graded into bleeding within the muscles and bleeding between the muscles (Fig 7), known respectively as intramuscular and intermuscular haematoma. However, in many instances both forms of muscle injury are found together.

One essential difference between the two types of injury is the speed of recovery in each case, for in intramuscular trauma the recovery rate can be two or three times longer than in intermuscular injury. It is thought that the escape of blood along the intermuscular fascia planes leads to a speedier repair and less adhesions and scar tissue.

Physiotherapy

Once the limb has been rested for approximately 48 hours physical therapy can begin in the injured limb. Let me point out from the outset that while a limb is being rested the other parts of the player's body must be exercised to maintain muscle bulk and improve blood flow. Thus he should attend for body-work the morning after injury.

But to return to the injured area. Static exercises designed to prevent atrophy of the tissues in the traumatised limb are performed at 48 hours. However, the injured limb must not be actively moved, and passive exercises must not produce pain. *During the early phase of physiotherapy, pain indicates further damage, and thus the exercises to that area should cease for another 24 hours when the situation is reappraised.*

The programme of static exercises, gentle passive exercises graduating to active exercises with support, then against gravity, and finally against the resistance of weights, may take 7–21 days, depending on the nature of the muscle injury. During this period the situation must be assessed daily at first and then on alternate days. Clearly this regime is only practicable when the trainer or physiotherapist works full-time at a club. In amateur teams the player should be seen at least on alternate days, initially, and then as often as the circumstances allow.

44

The following example relates to an injured Second Division forward, who sustained a direct blow to the quadriceps, and was diagnosed as having a predominately intermuscular injury.

Day 0: I.C.E., pain-killing and anti-inflammatory tablets (such as ibuprofen, aspirin, indomethacin).

Day 1 (Sunday morning at 9.00 a.m.). Crêpe and wool support removed and early localisation of haematoma and swelling seen. Commenced body and upper limb exercises, also resistance exercises to the uninjured limb. Told to repeat exercises in afternoon.

Day 2 (Monday at 9.30 a.m., afternoon 1.30 p.m., and 4.30 p.m.). Attends for remedial exercises to all limbs (except injured) and decides that being ill is more demanding physically than playing. Injured limb inspected and the swelling is just beginning to subside. Early wasting noted in quadriceps, especially vastus medialis muscle. Slight passive movements produce a pain-response, static exercises deferred for 24 hours.

Day 3 (Tuesday, same times). The injured area is less tender and early bruising has appeared. Gentle static exercises are begun with the trainer supporting the heel. Very little movement is allowed at the knee.

Day 4 (Wednesday, same times). Encouraging response to static exercises allows more knee flexion and early anti-gravity exercises (i.e. the leg is raised on its own without producing pain).

Day 5 (Thursday, 9.30 a.m., 1.30 p.m.). The player is now encouraged to carry out forty anti-gravity, straight-leg-raisings, beginning at five minutes to each hour. The bruising in the thigh is more marked, but the muscle is much less tender to deep palpation.

Day 6 (Friday, 9.30 a.m., 1.30 p.m.). The quadriceps bulk has begun to return and the player continues his exercises, supplemented by 5–10 lb. on each foot.

Day 7 (Saturday, 9.30 a.m.). Has almost a full range of knee

movements. Quadriceps bulk has almost reached normal proportions. Weights are increased to 20–25 lb. on the foot during
straight-leg-raising. Player watches first team match.

Day 9 (Monday 9.30 a.m.). Gentle jogging, crouching, wall-
exercises are commenced.

Day 10 (9.30 a.m.). Shoulder weights during squats (no more
than 40–60 lb.). gentle dead ball kicking begins.

Day 11. Improvement continues and pronounced fit for next
game, although two days of intensive field work remains to build
up stamina.

Please note that heat as short-wave diathermy and plaster have
not been used in this example, although they have their place
in certain muscle injuries.

*Massage of an injured area is never used. There is no evidence
it breaks down adhesions. Massage may also produce further
muscle damage and bone formation in the tissues.*

I know of one international player who was so pummelled
after every muscle injury that he developed scarring and later
calcification in the muscles.

Let us consider short-wave diathermy in muscle injuries.
Despite the rather technical name, S.W.D. means heat, and
heat increases blood flow by dilating the blood vessels. Therefore, as stated in Chapter 2, heating an area during the injury
phase only makes the swelling worse. Once the swelling has begun to subside then short periods of heating can be carried out,
with some reduction in pain and spasm. However, I have never
seen a properly controlled trial of the use of heat in sports
injuries, and it has never been adequately proved that heating
is greatly beneficial in promoting the repair of muscle injuries.
Trainers often heat when they can think of nothing else to do;
and basic rest and graduated therapy are forgotten.

Intramuscular injuries of the thigh usually respond in 10–20
days, while intermuscular injuries at the same site take between
8–15 days.

The recovery of a muscle injury has not taken place until:

full power;

extensibility;

range of joint movements; and

skill patterns have returned.

The ability of a muscle group to stretch to its fullest is vital for maximum power, e.g., the sprinter's crouch which stretches all key muscle groups and produces the powerful contraction necessary for a sudden burst. Without full stretching of the opposing muscles athletic performance falls.

Pulled Muscles

Indirect muscle injuries occur at the weak point of muscle/tendon (where the fibrous tissue leaves the muscle and is carried forwards into the tendon), ligament or periosteum (the fibrous skin around the bone). Such injuries are known as musculotendinous or musculo-periosteal tears.

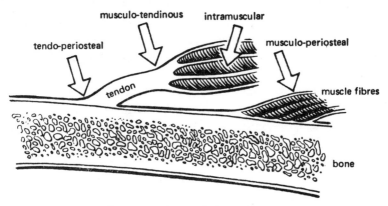

8. Insertions where pulled muscles occur.

The common pulled muscles of footballers, sprinters, hurdlers and jumpers are the hamstring group, the so-called pulled hamstring (although one of three muscles may be involved). Classically there is sudden pain in either the lateral hamstrings (the

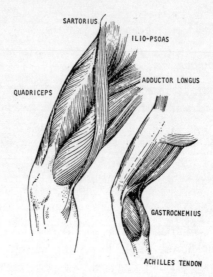

SARTORIUS

ILIO-PSOAS

ADDUCTOR LONGUS

QUADRICEPS

GASTROCNEMIUS

ACHILLES TENDON

9. Commonly pulled muscles of the lower limb.

biceps femoris) or the medial hamstrings (semimembranosus and semitendinosus) at their junction of muscle belly and tendon. In effect, the sudden unguarded strain on the muscle pulls the fibres out of their sockets in the tendon, with minimal bleeding and swelling.

On examination there is little to find except a markedly tender area at the tearing point. The diagnosis is made on the circumstances of injury – namely a sudden pain in the muscle, a dramatic cessation of activity and an inability to bring the injured limb into the follow-through position of hurdling i.e., stretching the hamstrings by raising the leg from the ground in a forward direction.

I recall being asked to see a member of the Kenyan Commonwealth team at the 1970 Commonwealth Games in Edinburgh, who, on easily taking the water-jump, suddenly developed a severe pain in the hamstrings and collapsed on the track. He had developed a tear at the musculo-tendinous junction in the biceps femoris muscle. He was also anxious to compete on the following day in the heats of another event, but was actively discouraged. It is not uncommon, even in the Olympics, to witness sprinters wearing uncouth, thick bandages around an injured thigh in an attempt to prevent further muscle injury. The hamstrings act vertically in the thigh, and no amount of strapping around these muscles will prevent their contraction. The only way to immobilise a hamstring is to place the pelvis and lower limb in a plaster, and that does not allow normal sitting never mind sprinting.

Much has been written on hamstring injuries, and if one believes the old saying that the more that is written about a subject the less is known about it, then one realises the complexity of treating hamstring injuries (and other pulled muscle syndromes). For the literature on this topic is exhaustive. It is important to realise that pulled muscles usually occur in tendons that cross two joint surfaces with opposing actions (for example the hamstrings extend the hip and flex the knee) or oppose more powerful muscle groups (for example the adductors at the groin balance the very powerful abductors of the hip). The resulting imbalance during activity causes the muscle to suddenly contract or relax insufficiently, and the fibres are torn.

Before the event the muscle groups should be stretched, gently but firmly, for about 20 minutes in the warm-up period. This procedure is far more beneficial to the athlete than running aimlessly around the track or jogging up or down on the spot. Once the hamstrings have been 'pulled' then all strenuous activity is usually 'out' for 6 weeks. In less severe cases, when all the player has felt is a faint niggle in the thigh, then remedial exercises to build up the surrounding muscles and gradual passive-elongation of the injured muscle will all aid recovery in 1–3 weeks. Steroid injections are almost useless in pulled muscle injuries, heat (in the later stages) gives some symptomatic relief, while ultrasound can be beneficial if the torn area is accurately localised. Like short-wave diathermy, it should be withheld until swelling or pain is subsiding.

To commence a stretching regime during the healing phase

will only invite recurrence. Once a hamstring injury has become chronic then the future is bleak for the player; there are few bites on the cherry in hamstring injuries.

Look for other pulled muscles in the region of the iliac crests of the pelvic rim (sartorius muscle), groin (adductor longus and ilio-psoas muscles) and the quadriceps of the thigh. (Chronic groin strain will be discussed in the next chapter). *Do not be misled by the shortage of signs after a pulled muscle injury, the pain and loss of function should give the game away.*

Stiffness

Stiffness is due to an accumulation of fluid within the muscle after strenuous exercise, and the frantic massaging of calf and thigh by the trainer after a hard 90 minutes of a cup-tie is designed to squeeze fluid back into the vessels of the legs. Too vigorous kneading of the muscles only makes the swelling worse.

In addition to gentle massage, the limb should be raised above heart level. This promotes venous return to the trunk. In the case of leg stiffness, the players should lie on the pitch with the leg elevated by the trainer and his assistants, and gravity will propel the tissue fluid down the limb. Gently moving the foot up and down will also help venous return. Despite stiffness and cramp in the World Cup Final of 1966 against Germany, the English players were able to raise their game in extra-time. It was an amazing sight to see the England players festooning the pitch, while the trainer and his assistants worked diligently to reduce muscle stiffness. Such prompt attention to detail can give a team that added advantage when the chips are down!

Should the muscle stiffness reach the proportions that it interferes with the blood supply to the muscle fibres, then cramp supervenes. A cramp of the abdominal muscles is referred to as 'the stitch'.

As a general rule fatigued players turn to a warm (or even hot) bath immediately after a match. This warmth will (of course) make stiffness worse. The heat of the bath increases the blood flow to the muscles, fluid pours out into the tissues and oedema increases.

The correct procedure is to warm down – something most players have never heard about! It means that after a match spend 5 or 10 minutes jogging, walking, gently stretching muscle groups (as in the warm up) and lying with the back to the floor or bench, with the legs raised from the ground. This procedure speeds up the fluid return from the legs. Then a coldish shower should be taken – the cold will help to close the dilated blood vessels and reduce further oedema.

Tendon Injury

Tendons are enormously strong since their function is to converge muscle pull into one narrow strip on the bone; in fact the forces which act across tendons can be as great as half a ton per square inch. Tendons contain special nerve endings which are designed to reflexly inhibit over-contraction, but tears do occur when co-ordination is impaired by fatigue or imbalanced skill.

Tendons consist of parallel bundles of collagen fibres which can be stretched or torn under extremes of movement. The sudden stubbing of the toes against a hard ground will forcibly stretch the extensor tendons on the anterior aspect of the ankle joint and a sprain results. When one examines sprained tendons during the course of an operation, minute tears or haemorrhages may be seen around or in the tendon bundles. But if the forces applied to the tendon are a little greater, as for example when two players collide in mid-air and one falls awkwardly to the ground with the weight of the other on top of his body, then the tendon may tear in part or completely.

Tendon tears are *partial,* or *complete,* and any tendon in the body can be torn. The commonest are the long head of biceps in the arm, the plantaris (a small accessory tendon) in the calf, the tendons of the shoulder (especially the supraspinatus) and the Achilles tendon at the heel.

When a tendon is ruptured there is little swelling apart from a localised swelling within the tendon sheaths (the fibrous covering around the tendon), and a creaking sensation on moving the affected parts (called crepitus and likened to the creaking of old leather). The swelling of the sheaths is often described as tendinitis, but true tendinitis is a chronic or over-use injury when the tendon is markedly damaged. When a tendon is badly torn (and this includes the occasional severe partial tear) then it must be repaired surgically and rested in plaster for 3–6 weeks. The Achilles tendon commonly ruptures with a snap, and there is an inability of the player to run or even waggle the foot.

The classical features of a tendon tear are:

pain over the torn area, radiating along the line of the muscle belly or tendon insertion;

loss of movement in the part supplied by the tendon;

a palpable gap at the torn area and a thickened area above or below the gap where the tendon ends have curled.

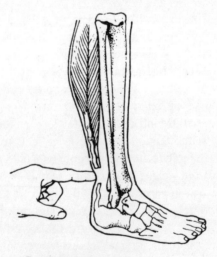

Ruptured Achilles tendon

10. Ruptured Achilles tendon.

I remember one footballer attending the Casualty Department convinced that he had been kicked on the calf, but on turning at the time noticed that the nearest player was at least 5 yards away. He had sustained a classical tear of the Achilles tendon, with a palpable gap just above the heal and weakness in pointing the foot downwards. The history of believing that someone has trodden on or kicked the calf region is quite common.

The rehabilitation after tendon injuries has to be planned and gradual, as after muscle injuries. Since collagen fibres take 3 weeks to become strong again, this is the minimum time to full recovery. If the tendon has to be repaired surgically then 6 weeks of immobilisation in a plaster is mandatory. Scarring around the healed tendon can be a nuisance, and bearing in mind that a repaired tendon may be only 70–80 per cent of its original strength, it is not hard to imagine that sporting performance falls and often the athlete has to abandon his career. However, Colin Cowdrey continued as a first-class cricketer following the repair of his torn Achilles tendon, and Uwe Seeler, West Germany, came back to re-appear in the World Cup finals in Mexico.

Ligament Injury

This is the commonest injury sustained by footballers, the most readily diagnosed and often the most perfunctorily treated. Like tendons, ligaments consist of collagen and elastic fibres with the former predominating. However, unlike tendons, the fibres are not bound in discreet bundles but fan out in intimate contact with the joint capsule; often ligaments are little more than thickening in the capsule along lines of force, such a condition occurs at the knee.

When a force is applied to a joint it first of all stretches the ligaments which act as a barrier to excess or abnormal movement. Should the force continue to act across the joint then the ligament becomes stretched, the minute fibres tear and a sprain results. Should the forces continue then the ligament becomes partially or completely torn.

53

Thus ligamentous injuries are:

sprain;

partial tear;

complete tear.

It is not unusual to tear one side of a joint and crush the other, as the diagram shows. Other structures, including the menisci (or cartilages) within the knee can be damaged at the same time. When a complete tear occurs in several ligaments of a joint or the capsule is unduly stretched, then a dislocation of the joint is found.

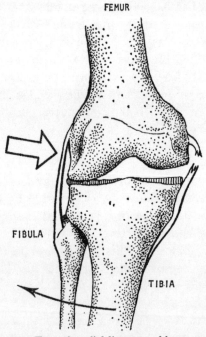

11. Tear of medial ligament of knee.

A sprain is easily diagnosed by tenderness over a ligament, slight swelling and loss of full movement in the joint. It is treated by rest, crêpe and wool or adhesive strapping.

However, a partial tear (when the signs are more severe and the ligament allows undue mobility at the joint) will need a plaster for 3 weeks, followed by intensive remedial exercises.

When ligament is completely torn the symptoms and signs are an exaggeration of the partial tear. A complete rupture demands surgical repair and a plaster for 3–6 weeks.

Although some professional footballers suffer from chronic stretching of the ligaments, especially around the knee and ankle, often it is imperative to ascertain if further acute stretching or tearing has occurred. When there is pain on moving the injured joint or effusion, then additional damage has been inflicted on those ligaments. It is no use the trainer thinking, 'Oh, that's only the give on his bad knee.' Joints weakened by ligamentous laxity are prone to repeated injury, especially around the medial ligament of the knee and the lateral ligament of the ankle.

Once a player has developed laxity of a ligament he will have to concentrate on muscle exercises to build up rock-hard muscles around the joint. These will compensate and allow peak performance. I have known international footballers with weak ligaments who turned in first-class performances weekly, and who could knock balls 30–40 yards with ease; totally relying on muscle tone to make up for their ligament instability.

It is an interesting fact that when one stands, one relies upon the congruity of bones and the tone in ligaments to keep upright. Muscle power plays little part. One can move the patella around while standing still, showing that the quadriceps are relaxed. However, during activity the muscles control joint movement, although the ligaments play their part. Footballers must have good muscle tone to protect their joints and ligaments from undue stretching and trauma. How common it is to see players with crêpe supports around the knee wholly confident that the joint will stand up to the stresses and strains of running. What they need is good muscle power, in this case a long period of quadriceps exercises.

The Medial Ligament of the Knee

The medial ligament of the knee is often torn by a hard tackle from the outside against the knee or an inside tackle on the ankle, thus forcing the leg away from the mid-line. In some cases the medial cartilage is torn at the same time. The player experiences immediate pain on the inside of the knee, and loss of movement. A careful examination indicates wobbling of the tibia on the femur. As explained, complete tears need surgical repair and plaster for 3–6 weeks. Static quadriceps exercises are commenced the next day, and body work is kept up during the immobilisation period.

Partial tears of the medial ligament often result in a chronic weakness of the inside of the knee (a once common injury in the old-fashioned winger, or hard-tackling half-back). Partial tears need plaster for 3–6 weeks.

Cruciate Damage in the Knee

The anterior cruciate may be torn when a player falls from a height, usually a corner, and the knee buckles up beneath his body forcing the femur backwards and the tibia forwards. Another injury situation consists of the player falling with another player across his thigh. As indicated by the arrows of force in the drawings, the anterior ligament is torn.

There is immediate pain in the knee and swelling (or effusion) rapidly occurs. Muscle spasm prevents the player from carrying on with the game and he may have to be 'stretchered off'. An examination of the knee reveals undue forward movement of the tibia on the femur.

Luckily, if there is only an isolated injury of the anterior cruciate then the quadriceps muscle can compensate and no operation is needed. A crêpe and wool bandage or plaster is applied to the knee, and quadriceps exercises begin. Usually the knee effusion persists for 2–4 weeks and during this period the player must use crutches and not walk on the knee. Once the swelling has subsided then quadriceps exercises begin in earnest, until the knee feels stable on standing and jogging.

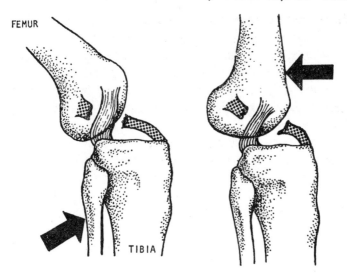

12 & 13. A rupture of the anterior cruciate ligament.

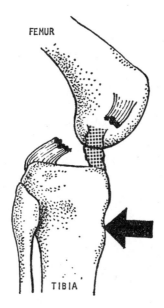

14. A rupture of the posterior cruciate ligament.

57

However, posterior cruciate tears are another matter!

Classically the goal situation is 'on' for the centre-forward with a 50/50 ball. The goalkeeper runs out to meet him, and falls across the on-rushing forward's leg as he tries to slip the ball under the keeper's body. There is a sudden heap of players, a tangle of arms and legs, and the forward emerges clutching his flexed knee.

Examination reveals pain on movement of the tibia backwards, and an effusion in the knee and in the space behind the knee (the popliteal fossa). Although surgical repair of the posterior cruciate has been regularly carried out, the results are not always of sufficient value to allow the player to return to soccer.

When both the anterior and posterior cruciates are torn, the knee is rendered very unstable, and often the medial cartilage and medial ligaments are torn. This injury always ends a foot-balling career.

The Ligaments of the Ankle

The ankle joint is really two joints balanced one upon the other (as the diagram shows) and to maintain stability of the bony parts there are numerous short, strong ligaments around it, attached chiefly to the tibia, fibula, talus and calcaneus. Some of these small ligaments are thickened, especially on the inner and outer aspects, and are called the medial and lateral ligaments of the ankle. Both are prone to injury in footballers. On occasions the ligaments tear and the bones are fractured and/or dislocated at the same time (a Pott's fracture).

Sprains of the capsule of the ankle are chiefly caused by tackles from behind, and depending on the direction of the tackle, the lateral ligament, anterior fibres of the medial ligament, or the anterior capsule are damaged, alone or in combination. Pain is localised along the torn ligament. Sprains of the ankle can be treated by strapping (from toe to knee) for 3–14 days, while tears need a plaster for 2–3 weeks. Should a tear of the lateral ligament be missed and not adequately treated then

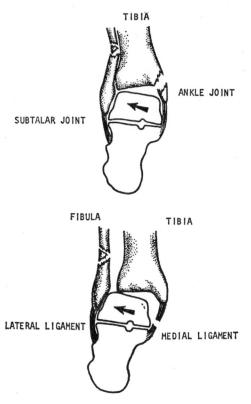

TIBIA

ANKLE JOINT

SUBTALAR JOINT

FIBULA   TIBIA

LATERAL LIGAMENT

MEDIAL LIGAMENT

15. A type of Pott's fracture of the ankle.

the fibres become stretched, and on running the ankle feels unstable and lets the player down.

Sprains of the Shoulder Region

Sprains of the shoulder region are common in goalkeepers repeatedly reaching for high balls and falling on the shoulder with low dives, especially at opponents' feet.

The ligaments retaining the clavicle (collar-bone) to the acromial process of the scapula can be stretched leading to a weakness of the shoulder, and players often complain of a dull ache at the tip of the shoulder while practising.

59

Football Fitness and Injuries

If the weakness at the acromio-clavicular junction is quite marked and the clavicle forms a prominence over the acromion, then two or three weeks of rest, strapping over the outer end of the clavicle and exercises to strengthen the deltoid and pectoral muscles will cure this condition.

When the arm is abruptly forced downwards, as occurs when a goalkeeper is attempting to punch a high ball and the opposing centre-forward collides with the outstretched arm, the small stabilising muscle of the shoulder (the supraspinatus) may be torn leading to acute shoulder pain and an inability to hold the arm at 20° from the trunk. If the arm is supported through an

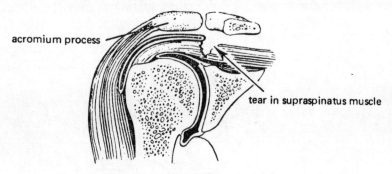

16. One of the common injuries in the rotator muscles of the shoulder.

arc of 30° by the trainer, then the large, fleshy deltoid takes over and the arm can be lifted from the body. Because the action of the deltoid can mask the weakness in the supraspinatus muscle, weakness during the first stage of shoulder movement (0–20°) must be looked for carefully. Complete rupture of the supraspinatus requires surgical suture, but partial tears heal in 3–4 weeks with the arm rested in a sling.

This may be an opportune time to explain the difference between a sling and a collar-and-cuff.

A sling supports the shoulder, while a collar-and-cuff allows the elbow to hang free and thus there is a drag on the shoulder. A sling is used for shoulder injuries, a collar-and-cuff is employed when the humerus is fractured and gravity is needed to straighten out the bone ends.

Cartilage Damage in the Knee

The cartilages within the knee are the bête noir of footballers, the site of the injury which most players fear, accept and talk about. The frequency of cartilage damage in the knee is often exaggerated, and players talk about it without really knowing the most elementary facts.

There are two types of cartilage injury, *the acute,* and *the chronic.* The acute injury has a classical onset. The player is darting in from the wing, trying to round a defender when he is suddenly checked either by the opposition or by heavy ground conditions. At this instant (on an action replay) the player's body is over a flexed knee, the knee is twisted slightly and the cartilages are taking up their normal position in the centre of the joint. The player attempts to accelerate forwards on his trapped leg while the thigh straightens on the knee. Under normal conditions the cartilages would rapidly move away from the advancing femur. But if the small retaining ligaments are weakened or the movement is very rapid, the cartilages, usually the medial, becomes torn and the knee locks or gives way. On other occasions the player is barged or tackled heavily from the side and the twisting motion imparted to the knee tears the cartilage as the knee bends.

The chronic injury is usually accompanied by several weeks or months of aching (on one side of the joint, or a dull internal joint pain) with some instability on running and climbing stairs. Initially the aching signifies stretching of the small ligaments that retain the cartilages at the outskirts of the knee, eventually the cartilages take up a more central position and a sudden twist or knock tears a small area. Repeated small tears during the season lead to a locking episode when the player cannot straighten or fully bend his knee.

Strangely enough, this is one of the few soccer injuries which can occur in the dressing-room, the knee suddenly locking as the player straightens up from tying his boots. I have seen this occur on two occasions.

I recall watching a trainer in the World Cup of 1966 vainly trying to reduce a locked knee on the field at Roker Park, while the Italian and Chilean teams looked on. The trainer

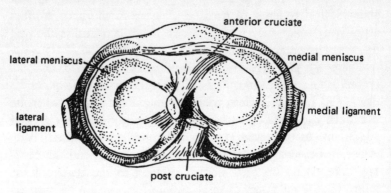

17. Knee joint from above.

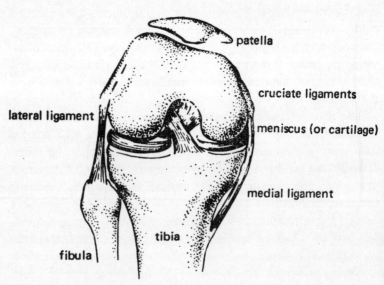

18. Knee joint from the front.

managed to straighten the knee to about 30° from the horizontal and then proceeded to wrap a large crêpe bandage around the leg. The player hobbled on the wing for some time before coming off.

Even if the knee can be reduced into a straight position after a cartilage tear, the player should not be allowed to continue playing, as ligaments may be stretched and damaged, and effusion made worse. Sometimes the club doctor can reduce the torn cartilage without an anaesthetic, but usually muscle spasm precludes such an event.

Many sportsmen have had their sporting career ruined by trying to persevere with a torn cartilage. Repeatedly unlocking the knee is dangerous therapy since it risks damage to the important cruciates and medial ligaments, and also the early onset of osteoarthritis. Damaged cartilages require excision, and if the quadriceps exercises are begun the same day, then the player will maintain his muscle bulk and be fit for playing in 4–8 weeks.

The Quadriceps Muscle

Because the powerful thigh muscle (on the anterior aspect) is a four-part muscle it is called the quadriceps, and this is the key to recovery in all knee joint pathology. Good quadriceps power will compensate for weak knee ligaments.

If one inspects the inner aspect of the knee closely one will see the bulky fibres of vastus medialis at their attachment into the inner border of the patella. These fibres rapidly disappear after knee injuries, leaving a floppy knee cap and unstable knee. *The key to successful recovery after knee injuries resides in strong and healthy quadriceps, especially the vastus medialis.* Trainers, encourage players to carry out regular quadriceps exercises, have weighted boots (10,20,30-plus lb.) for resistance exercises and straight-leg raising, always watch the vastus medialis for early signs of wasting, make players work hard after knee joint injuries with straight-leg raising, 40 times each hour, beginning at 5 minutes to the hour, and lasting 5–10 minutes.

63

Good quadriceps power helps to keep footballers knees in good condition, and prolongs active life!

Skin Care

The skin is the barrier between the germ-laden outside environment and the germ-free inner world of the human frame. Players can loose more time from skin ailments than from muscle injuries.

All players must be immunised against tetanus. The organisms of tetanus are found in all soils, and despite antibiotics an infection often proves fatal. Booster doses of tetanus toxoid are given every 3–5 years.

All wounds must be thoroughly cleaned with a very mild antiseptic (strong antiseptics kill the delicate tissues, and this dead area acts as a centre for the germs to multiply, while pastes often contain a multitude of bacteria, as I mentioned (in Chapter 2) and covered with a sterile dressing or mercurochrome solution. If a laceration is contaminated with grass and soil then the wound may need surgical excision. Gas gangrene germs can lurk in soil fragments. Vaseline impregnated dressings (tulle gras) can be used at friction areas such as the inner thigh or buttock.

Antibiotic sprays are never a substitute for the efficient cleaning and sterile dressings, although they are an additional safeguard if one follows the above regimen.

Small lacerations over the face require special adhesive tape sutures, but larger cuts need stitching. *All lacerations are potentially dangerous and need careful inspection to see if tendons, ligaments, nerves, blood vessels, bones and joints are involved.*

Footballers are prone to fungal infection between the toes and in the groin, and the fungus may be transmitted in the communal bath. Antifungal creams, supplied by the doctor, are needed to eradicate the skin irritation, but often the fungus is passed round the club in strict rotation, and all personnel need treatment at once since they may be potential carriers.

Finally, the toe nails must be clean, cut correctly and not broken so that jagged edges lie below the nail folds. If the skin on the toe is compressed by too tightly-fitting boots, and infection supervenes, an in-growing toe nail can result and may be troublesome to cure. Players may miss up to 8 weeks with an in-growing toe nail.

Soft tissue must be cared for in a meticulous, fanatical way, and the player's career will be prolonged for many years, to the benefit of all concerned.

Chapter Four

Soft Tissue Injuries – Chronic

Chronic injuries of the soft tissues can begin as an acute injury, and because of inadequate therapy become chronic; or in other instances the injury simply appears out of the blue, and over a period of matches becomes worse and worse. *An inadequately treated chronic injury will spell the end of a playing career.*

Every sportsman, from the top Olympic athlete to the part-time footballer has certain limitations in performance that eventually determine his standard of competition. It may be heart or lungs, or muscle power, or nerve co-ordination; however, in some players the limiting factors are the soft tissues. For example, why all footballers do not suffer from recurring Achilles tendinitis is not known, the unlucky few may have been born with a slightly abnormal tendon, or have poor running style and posture. Whatever the factors involved, there are certain players who will never make the top grade because they are not suited for top-class sport, whether it is due to eyesight, heart, lungs, muscles, tendons, etc. These players must be told, and directed towards a sport they can become proficient in. It is useless to continue treatment of a sportsman beyond a certain point when he is suffering from a recurrent injury.

The best way to treat chronic injuries is to prevent their occurrence by strict attention to acute injuries, and never rush a player back to match play before he is 100 per cent fit.

The villain of the piece is 'scar tissue', that dense, haphazard arrangement of collagen fibres which binds down tendons, muscles, nerves, and other structures. Once the scar tissue contracts the involved tissues are strangled, leading to painful, limited movements.

The essence of treatment is to limit the formation of scar tissue by rest and then stretch the scarring by graduated exercises once the collagen is strong. In rare circumstances, for example adhesions in a joint, the scar tissue can be torn by manipulation, and the process of rest and exercises begin again under strict medical supervision.

Peritendinitis

Peritendinitis is an inflammation of long standing around tendons, which reduces their mobility and produces painful, uncoordinated movements of the areas involved.

It can be due to:

Simple over-use injuries e.g., golfer's or tennis elbow,

partial, but repeated, tears e.g., in the Achilles tendon,

incomplete healing after an acute tear, e.g., groin strain in the thigh.

However, it is often very difficult to determine the exact origins of the injury, which may begin insidiously and be ignored for some while, in the belief that it will fade away.

Although each injury will be dealt with in turn, the fundamental principles of *rest, graduated therapy and alteration in style* are familiar to them all.

Chronic Shoulder Injuries

After a dislocation or fracture around the shoulder the athlete may develop a painful arc of movement with limited mobility. Should the capsule of the shoulder joint be severely scarred then all sporting pursuits involving this joint will be permanently impaired. No amount of manipulation of the shoulder will restore normal movement, especially if there has been a fracture into the joint (an intra-articular fracture). However, part of the capsule of the shoulder joint consists of small muscles (including

67

the supraspinatus) and tearing of the muscle fibres can restrict rotary function and abduction of the arm. Then the condition is referred to as supraspinatus tendinitis, or becomes a frozen shoulder.

A frozen shoulder may arise without any obvious cause, or after injections in the arm (e.g. tetanus inoculation), illness, or injury in the shoulder or arm. All ranges of movement are severely limited, and in some instances there is only a jog of motion. The condition may persist for 6–9 months, but usually responds to heat, physiotherapy, anti-inflammatory tablets and steroid injections.

Calcification and degeneration in the small muscles and tendons around the joint is sometimes found in athletes, and the supraspinatus tendon irritates the subacromial bursa (see figure 19) leading to a painful arc of shoulder movements at 50° of abduction. If calcification is marked, it can be removed surgic-

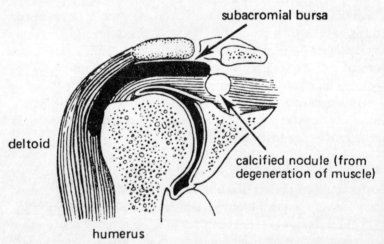

subacromial bursa

deltoid

calcified nodule (from degeneration of muscle)

humerus

calcified nodule in supraspinatus muscle, has caused—by friction—a swelling of the subacromial bursa

19. Calcified nodule in supraspinatus muscle has caused, by friction, a swelling of the subacromial bursa.

ally, otherwise the treatment is the same as for frozen shoulder.

Tendinitis of the biceps tendon follows unaccustomed use, as for example tennis or golf (often called golfer's shoulder). The shoulder looks normal but tenderness is found in the bicipital groove on the anterior aspect of the arm. Rest and local heat usually cures this condition, but a partial rupture of the biceps muscle could be easily missed.

Tennis Elbow

This condition is not exclusively found in tennis stars, but is often described as 'do-it-yourself elbow' because of its frequent association with painting and decorating. Goalkeepers who have their hands thrust continually back (hyperextended at the wrist) due to faulty catching technique may suffer from pain at the insertion of the extensor tendons on the outer aspect of the elbow. A tender spot is found over this outer aspect of the humerus, and a handshake which forces the wrist towards ulna causes pain. Usually tennis elbow settles with rest and steriod injections, rarely a plaster is needed.

Sometimes a tenosynovitis of the wrist tendons accompanies tennis elbow, and responds to a similar regime of treatment.

A special chronic thickening is found above the radial styloid at the wrist, especially in goalkeepers. It is called De Quervain's syndrome. A palpable, thickened area with local swelling is felt over the involved tendons, and surgical release of the tendons offers a speedy cure.

Groin Strain

One of the commonest recurrent problems in soccer is 'groin strain'. The commonly affected tendon is the adductor longus at its insertion into the pubic bone of the pelvis. However, other tendons can be strained in the groin, including the origin of rectus femoris above the hip, the sartorious at the iliac spine, and the ilio-psoas muscle. In all cases the initial injury is the same, namely an unguarded movement at the hip in a fatigued player which tears the muscle at the insertion into bone or tendon. A small amount of internal bleeding is produced, but the swelling is not felt on examination. Pain and loss of function are marked, and the player has difficulty in stretching the lower limb in relation to the trunk.

There are no short cuts in the treatment of groin strain, and a hasty return to match play or full training invites recurrence.

The diagnosis is made by tenderness over the tendon insertion (usually the adductor longus muscle) and pain on attempting to run, jump or, in severe cases, walk. If the player is asked to push the leg inwards with resistance (i.e. push the inside of the foot against a wall) a sharp pain is often felt running down the inside of the thigh.

Groin strains often take 2–4 weeks to recover depending on their severity and number of previous attacks. The initial treatment is rest from training (no strapping is of any value) and analgesic tablets like Ibuprofen ('Brufen'), soluble aspirin or Indomethacin. After 3–7 days depending upon the symptoms the player begins Short Wave Diathermy and graduated exercises, although straight leg raising exercises are forbidden until the leg can be raised passively (by the trainer) without producing pain. Once thigh extension exercises are painless, straight running can be commenced, with eventual jumping, dead-ball kick-from hands and then ground, until the final remedial exercises are carried out at speed, in the sand-pit and up the hard steps of the stand. If the player is proficient in these tests then he can return to match-play, but not until!

Chronic adductor tendinitis, although common in horse-riders (where the tendon becomes calcified) and swimmers (with a poor leg action), is rare in footballers. For this refractory condition a manipulation under general anaesthetic has been advocated, but the results may be disappointing.

Occasionally there is a tender area over the greater trochanter of the femur (the prominent bone on the upper, outer thigh) which is due to an inflamed bursa. The area can be injected with hydrocortisone, and the condition usually subsides (*trochanteric bursitis*).

Recurrent Pulled Hamstrings

This injury which produces pain during the follow-through phase of sprinting is difficult to treat once established. Tearing of the muscle fibres can occur at several points along the hamstring muscles, and pain is typically felt when the hamstrings are stretched, especially on sitting down. A sharp pain may also radiate down the leg.

The treatment is the same as for recurrent groin strain.

Chronic Pain in the Knee

The knee is by far and away the most complex joint in the body, with several types of movement possible at the same time. There are three compartments: the inner (or medial) articulation between femur and tibia, the outer (or lateral) articulation between femur and tibia, and the articulation between patella and femur.

The inner and outer articulations are in turn divided into two by the cartilages (or menisci), while the cruciate ligaments cross the joint from front to back (see Fig. 18).

In a young player pain in the knee can be due to fraying or tearing of the cartilages, or softening of the cartilage on the back of the patella. Occasionally a loose piece of bone or cartilage causes locking and aching within the knee. Rarely, the fatty pad which separates the patella tendon from the tibia gets nipped, and a tender area is found below the knee cap.

Goalkeepers who repeatedly fall on their knees may develop a bursa in front of the patella tendon (rather like 'housemaid's' or 'parson's knee'. Another swelling which presents at the level of the joint line (nearly always the lateral) is a cyst of the cartilage.

There are other swellings around the knee. A lump in the popliteal fossa is called a popliteal bursa and is usually related to wearing in the knee joint; but a cyst under the semimembranosus tendon does not communicate with the knee joint and presents as a small nodule at the insertion of the semimebranosus muscle.

71

Football Fitness and Injuries

Partial tears in the quadriceps extensor tendon or straining in the patellar tendon can give rise to a dull ache around the knee, especially after dead-ball practice.

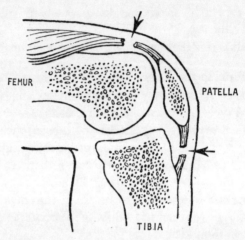

20. Tears in the extensor muscles and patellar ligament.

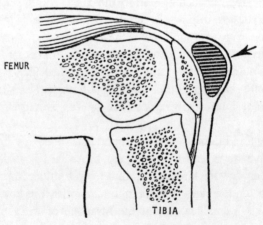

21. Pre-patellar bursitis.

In older sportsmen a slight amount of osteoarthritis is found in all three compartments, especially when the knee has been subjected to repeated injury; or when ligamentous or cartilaginous damage has been ignored. The hyaline articular cartilage becomes rough, fibrillated and thinned, then pieces may flake off. The bone beneath the damaged cartilage becomes sclerosed and forms tiny cysts. At the non-pressure areas the cartilage proliferates and calcifies, forming spiky nodules known as osteophytes which are obvious on X-ray. Excess fluid may be found in the joint, which becomes painful and thickened to the touch. With marked osteoarthritis the player has to give up his career. However, many footballers continue with mild osteoarthritic symptoms for years and reach international levels.

Chronic weakness in the cruciates and medial and lateral ligaments can give rise to an aching, unstable knee which does not respond to quadriceps exercises. These exercises should be used for several weeks until a final decision is made whether or not the player should continue his career. Most of the other conditions causing knee pain require medical advice and possible surgical correction. Offending cartilages need immediate excision.

Achilles Tendinitis

Although thickening can occur in the Achilles tendon due to over-use, many cases are due to partial tears in the tendon which never heal properly, and at operation the Achilles tendon is found to be degenerate. A sudden tearing of the Achilles tendon requires surgical suture and plaster for 6 weeks, but the function of the tendon may be permanently impaired (see Chapter 2).

The treatment for mild Achilles strain consists of rest in strapping or plaster, with short wave diathermy and analgesics. Graduated exercises are begun as soon as the player can stand on his toes without discomfort. However, jumping and sprinting are forbidden until the player can run smoothly and support weights

73

on his shoulders during squatting. Achilles tendon trouble usually takes 2–3 weeks to settle down.

Attention to the type of footwear a player uses is never more important than in the case of Achilles tendinitis. The current craze for high heels in men (promoted by the miniscule pop singers of today) leads to chronic shortening of the Achilles tendon, so that when the player wears flat plimsoles in the gym, the Achilles tendon is stretched compared to its 'normal' range of movement. Then they wonder why their Achilles tendons are aching! Incidently a player with ankle trouble (and this includes Achilles tendinitis) should be discouraged from training on hard tracks and wooden gym floors. He also should protect his heels with sorbo rubber insoles, and wear a slightly raised heel on the affected side.

Although the surgical stripping of the thickened sheath of the Achilles tendon may be carried out, the condition of the tendon may obviate against further sport, especially if there are large areas of degenerate collagen.

Shin Soreness
An aching sensation across the front of the leg to the ankle can be due to several conditions. An over-use of the anterior tibial muscles may be found after numerous cross-country runs. The repeated activity of the muscles leads to swelling within the leg fascia, and a dull pain becomes apparent after 1–2 miles. Another form of shin soreness occurs when there are fatigue fractures in the tibia or fibula, as outlined in Chapter 5.

The immediate treatment of shin soreness resides in rest and graduated exercises to build up the tibial muscles without causing too much hypertrophy. Often the conditions recurs, and an obligatory rest period of 3–6 months may be necessary to allow the condition to settle down. This rest period is best taken during the close season. Multiple subperiosteal haematomas give an irregular feel to the anterior surface of the tibia but are of no importance (footballer's shin).

Chronic Ligamentous Injury, including the Ankle

Acute sprains are common in athletes but rarely does the condition become recurrent unless there is a major tear in the ligament, defective motion of the bone (as for example after a poorly united fracture) or when there is poor muscle tone and control.

The ligaments of the shoulder and knee occasionally give rise to chronic, painful over-use lesions; but the ligaments of the ankle are commonly the site of recurrent strain.

The importance of the many small ligaments of the ankle in retaining the balance of the individual while running has been mentioned. Incorrect running style, repeated tackling, or fractures and dislocations around the ankle can lead to stretching of the ankle ligaments at the ankle or subtalar joints.

The ankle is one of the few joints which can be strapped and still allow activity. Unfortunately this privilege is abused on too many occasions, with the ultimate result of lateral or medial ligament weakness.

As the ligaments become stretched the ankle becomes more unstable and thus more liable to spraining. It is a vicious circle!

The circle can only be broken by adequate rest after an ankle sprain (1–3 weeks depending on the severity), with partial tears of the ligaments being immobilised in plaster for up to 4 weeks. A complete rupture may take 3–6 weeks to heal.

Chronic weakness of the lateral ligament may respond to an operation designed to strengthen the weakness using the available lateral malleolus and tendons. Treatment designed to strengthen the medial (or deltoid) ligament of the ankle by operative means is not so successful.

Acute tenosynovitis occurs around the ankle, usually in the tendons on the front of the joint. The area becomes puffy and tender due to swelling in the tendon sheaths but settles with rest, strapping and hydrocortisone. However, chronic thickening around the tendons needs prolonged rest, heat and physiotherapy. Footballer's ankle is due to repeated small tears in the anterior aspect of the ankle joint from dead-ball kicking and shooting. The many capsular scars produced become calcified and small spicules of bone are found at the insertion of the joint capsule into the bone. The player usually complains of a dull aching around the ankle, worse after use. The treatment of this condition is rest, manipulation and occasional excision of the bony lumps.

However, it must be pointed out that most professional footballers have spicules of bone around the ankle and never complain of any trouble. It is easy for the unwary, on looking at an ankle X-ray, to incriminate these tiny spicules of bone when a player complains of ankle pain. However, other joint trouble must be excluded.

In football the ankle is particularly vulnerable from sliding tackles or a 'clash of feet'. The anterior fibres of the lateral ligament are torn with this injury; while the posterior fibres of the lateral ligament may be torn when the opposing player's boot comes through in a tackle from behind. Thus, the trainer must be diligent in his approach to ankle injuries so that a potentially easily treatable condition does not become a chronic, incurable one.

Any joint that is repeatedly injured suffers from multiple small bleeds within the joint, and eventually the lining tissue of the joint (the synovial layer) becomes packed with iron pigments, thickened, and unable to remove the fluid from within the joint. The player has a painful, slightly swollen joint with a marked limitation of movement. In other circumstances the joint develops small hard ganglia at the site of degeneration within the ligament. In both these instances the ganglia or the thickened synovial layer may require surgical excision. The prognosis after ganglia resection is excellent, although after the latter operation (synovectomy) there may be impaired function. I have known, however, a professional player return to full playing capacity in the English League after a synovial resection of the ankle.

Many other small ligaments in the hands and feet may become strained but rarely do they progress to chronic trouble, apart from the chronic ligament strain of the thumb in goalkeepers. The joint can be stabilised before playing with a plaster (sticky) thumb spica.

Painful Thighs

This condition warrants mention on its own, not because there is anything particular in repeated, small, acute muscle haematomas in this region, but because there is a considerable likelihood that inadequate treatment will result in calcification and later ossification in the thigh muscles. This crippling condition is known as myositis ossificans.

Vigorous massage of the thigh muscles after a haematoma, or a persistance of the footballer in playing, may precipitate this complication. It begins as a deep-seated thickening in the thigh, and over a few weeks becomes obvious as a palpable, hard lump in the quadriceps muscle.

An astute trainer treats all quadriceps bleeds with care, by avoiding undue heating, massage and overactivity at too early a stage. Once the bony area has become established an operation may be employed to remove the bony mass, but the residual scarring in the muscles can end the playing career.

In some instances the cause of calcification may be unknown, and be due to some local abnormality in the thigh.

Chronic Back and Neck Strain

Everyone suffers from backache and footballers are no exception! Most cases of backache in athletes are due to minor strains in the small ligaments and muscles of the lumbar spine, although a prolapse of the intervertebral disc is occasionally found. Mild backache responds to rest, analgesics, heat and graduated spinal exercises. When symptoms of sciatica are found in association with lumbar pain, then the diagnosis is almost certainly due to a slipped disc. Rarely these symptoms can be caused by congenital bony abnormalities. Sometimes a manipulation relieves backache. However, it may be necessary to remove the bulging disc if the symptoms are severe or if the nerves in the back, supplying the leg, are being compressed leading to calf and thigh weakness and wasting. Players can return to training in 6–12 weeks following a back operation (laminectomy) depending upon the severity of the initial symptoms and the magnitude of the operation.

The onset of lumbar disc pain may be gradual or sudden. When the onset is gradual, there are intermittent attacks of backache lasting for 1–3 weeks, with eventual sciatic radiation. Over 3–5 years the symptoms gradually get worse and the player may feel he is walking on cotton-wool, or he may notice that the muscles in his legs look thinner or feel weaker.

The sudden onset lumbar disc occurs after a heavy fall or when doing something simple, like tying up the boot-laces or pulling on the sock with support from only one leg. In each instance the back is acutely flexed and the sudden pain may lock the patient in a stooping position. Heat applied to the lumbar area helps to relieve the muscle spasm and allow the player to lie down on a firm mattress. Medical advice should be sought.

Pain over the side of the neck and shoulder is often referred to as brachial neuralgia, and if often caused by minor sprains or disc trouble in the neck (or cervical) region. The condition remits with heat and analgesics. Rarely the pain radiates down the arm to the hand. Then physiotherapy and manipulation of the neck may be indicated.

There is no doubt that once a chronic soft tissue injury becomes established it can occupy a great deal of the trainer's time and patience. It is quite easy to 'lay the blame on the players' shoulders', especially when they resort to chronic injuries as an excuse for loss of form. However, no player should develop a chronic injury from an acute injury if the latter is correctly treated, while the gradual onset over-use injury should be nipped in the bud.

One can only reiterate: Never rush a player back to training or match play until he is fit, feels fit, and you are happy with the performance.

Chapter Five

Fractures and Dislocations

Fractures and dislocations are the most serious of complications found in sports medicine, and associated with long periods of immobility and high player-wastage. However, even the most serious of fractures (a fractured femur) can have a successful outcome as shown by the former Leeds player Bobby Collins.

Before continuing with this Chapter it is prudent to recall the signs and symptoms of a fracture and dislocation as outlined in Chapter 2. *Every trainer must be familiar with the presentation of fractures and dislocation. If in doubt treat an area as fractured until medical advice or an X-ray proves otherwise.*

I have known trainers demanding that players jog around on injured limbs to see if they could run off the pain. Undue movement at a fracture site can easily lead to a broken skin and the complications of a compound fracture (see Chapter 2).

Whenever a fracture occurs in a limb it is wise to assess the state of the circulation and nerves below the damaged area. A pink, warm skin with a good pulse denotes an adequate circulation; a mottled, bluish, swollen limb with poor pulses means an impaired vascular flow. Undue pain in a fracture area with weakness of movement down the limb and areas of numbness or tingling may indicate that the nerves are being severely compressed by the fracture or the swelling. In both types of fracture medical advice should be sought urgently, preferably the player taken straight to hospital.

Simple fractures may have dire consequences. For example an isolated rib fracture can penetrate the lung, liver or spleen; while a crack fracture of the pelvis may be associated with injury to the bladder outlet (the urethra). Also, fractures may extend into the joint (intra-articular) and the resulting incongruity of the joint surfaces lead to painful movement and stiffness.

Fractures may be divided into:

Simple or closed;

Open or compound.

When the fracture is compound, cover the wound. with a sterile cloth. Both of the above forms of fracture may be divided into various types depending upon the *pattern of fracture:*

comminuted fractures, when the bone is broken into three or more parts;

impacted fractures, when one fragment is driven into the other and no abnormal mobility found;

greenstick fractures occur in children when only one side of the bone is broken;

crush fractures occur in the spinal column, and the bones are squashed;

spiral and transverse fractures relate to the description of the damage produced;

fatigue (or stress) fractures occur without obvious injury;

pathological fractures are found in diseased bones. This type of fracture is very rare in athletes.

The initial treatment of all fractures is by correct splinting (as described in Chapter 2). Medical advice is needed to perform reduction and splinting. Minor fractures in non-weight-bearing bones can be treated by crêpe or adhesive strapping (e.g. thumb phalanges, big toe, fibula shaft) but most fractures need immobilisation in plaster, and some need internal fixation with metallic screws or plates.

Dislocations require immediate splinting and reduction in hospital, after an X-ray has confirmed that no bones are broken.

Skull Fractures

When a player receives a blow on the skull and a boggy swelling (which is a haematoma beneath the scalp) follows, it could indicate a fractured skull, although the player need not have been knocked out. The importance of skull fractures resides in the fact that any bleeding either from the fracture area or from the blood vessels within the skull can compress the delicate brain tissue. That is why no player who has been knocked out should be allowed to return to the match, for exercise will increase blood flow and the amount of bleeding.

All fractures of the skull must be observed for possible brain injury. Fractures above the ear, caused by a blow on the temporal region, may cause tearing of the middle meningeal artery or vein and an extradural haemorrhage. The diagnosis is by swelling and bruising above the ear, a short period of concussion followed by a lucid period when the player may act normally, later becoming confused, irritable and then unconscious as bleeding accumulates within the skull and compresses the brain. The pupils become irregular and dilated.

Always beware of a confused player in the dressing-room with a bruise on the temporal region.

Fractures above the nose (frontal region) may break a fine bone inside the skull and allow clear cerebrospinal fluid (like pure spring water) to escape from the nose; or it may be mixed with a slight quantity of blood. The player must on no account breath deeply or blow his nose as bacteria can be forced into the skull through the damaged area, thus risking meningitis. Obviously such a serious condition warrants hospital admission.

A black eye appearing some hours after a head injury, with no damage to the skin around the eye, and with a flame-shaped haemorrhage beneath the conjunctiva may indicate a fracture of the base of the skull.

Bleeding from the ear, if derived from a torn ear drum or damaged outer ear, will clot; if mixed with cerebrospinal fluid it continues to drip as rather watery-blood. These features indicate a fracture of the middle fossa of the base of the skull.
The cardinal features of a head injury are:

unconsciousness;

confusion, disorientation, irritability (behaving as if drunk, or showing aggressive personality out of character with normal manner);

headaches (pounding, worse on stooping or coughing);

vomiting.

When in doubt about a head injury always seek medical advice.

Facial Fractures

This area of the body can produce some very complex fractures which require immediate expert attention to prevent deformity, and poor cosmetic results. Blows to the nose can fracture the nasal bones or cartilages. Heavy bleeding may require a nasal pack with adrenaline solution and tube gauze. Any displacement of the nose requires surgical correction, but some Casualty Departments prefer to wait for 3–5 days and assess the degree of cosmetic deformity when the swelling has subsided. Players can return to football in 2–4 weeks after having the nose straightened. However, badly displaced fractures may necessitate a longer time off.

Blows above the nose may cause an abrasion of the cornea, with a feeling of grittiness in the eye; or they may produce a detachment of the retina or vitreous haemorrhage with a resulting loss in vision. All three conditions require hospital care.

Foreign bodies, such as pieces of mud or grass, are best removed from the eye with lavage with warm, sterile water. If the foreign body becomes trapped under the upper eyelid, then the lid can be bent over a sterile fine wooden spatula by gently lifting the eyelashes in an upward direction.

Double vision can result from a blow on the head and a mild

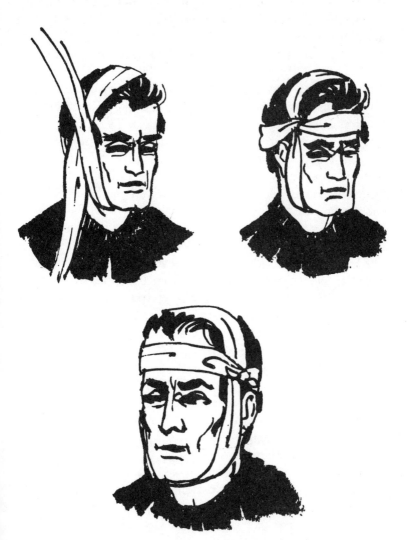

22. Methods of applying a face support.

head injury, or from damage to the soft tissues around the eye, especially if part of the floor of the eye socket (the malar or cheek bone) is fractured. Such a fracture occurs when there is a clash of heads at a corner. The diagnosis depends upon flattening of the cheek, numbness of the face, difficulty in opening the mouth, and double vision. This fracture needs an operation to allow the jaw to operate normally and to correct the numbness and double vision. Players usually are fit within 4–6 weeks.

Fractures of the mandible are caused by a direct blow on the jaw, and teeth may be knocked out at the same time. The player experiences pain over the jaw, difficulty in speaking and swallowing, and there is blood-stained saliva. *The trainer should cover any laceration on the face (or scalp) with a sterile dressing, and apply a supportive bandage.* The diagram indicates the common, and easily applied, jaw and face supportive bandage. Dental wiring is performed in hospital and the player may be out of action for 2–3 months.

Sometimes the blow on the jaw causes it to dislocate, especially if the mouth is open at the time of impact. The jaw is tilted towards one side, saliva dribbles down the chin and a hollow is felt in front of the ear. Reduction can be performed by pressing with padded thumbs on the lower molar teeth and rotating the chin forwards. An anaesthetic is usually needed, and the player wears a support on the chin for 2–4 weeks.

Fractures of the spine

Although common in horse-riders and jockeys, fractures of the spine are very rare in soccer players. Dislocations do occur in the cervical spine, which is the most mobile area, and occasionally in the thoracic spine. The signs of spinal damage have been referred to in Chapter 2.

The most important feature of any spinal damage is coincidental injury to the spinal cord and resulting muscle weakness and sensory nerve damage.

When the trainer suspects a spinal injury, the less the player is handled and moved, the better. Transport the injured person on a firm surface, e.g. a strong stretcher with a good canvas, or, in an emergency, a wooden board or door. If such equipment is not to be found, then it is occasionally justified to roll the patient gently on to a doubled-blanket for transportation. The player is transported supine with the head to one side if vomiting occurs. However, the head must not be moved around when the cervical spine is damaged. Transport the player with care.

The commonest injury in soccer players is a crush fracture of the vertebra, usually the lumbar, when a sudden, sharp pain is found in the back. The spinal cord is rarely damaged, and this fracture needs 2–3 weeks of bed rest, or plaster or spinal support if troublesome. Within 6–8 weeks the bone is healed and soccer can begin again.

Fractures of the Shoulder

The clavicle is the commonest long bone to fracture, usually due to a fall on the outstretched hand. Since this bone lies directly under the skin the deformity can be seen and felt. The treatment consists of a figure-of-eight bandage and a sling for 3–4 weeks, then mobilisation and training can commence. There are usually no after-effects.

A dislocation can be found at the acromioclavicular joint at the tip of the shoulder, and the clavicle comes to lie over the acromial process of the scapula. The precipitating cause is a heavy fall on to the shoulder. Goalkeepers are prone to this disorder. Although a simple injury to treat by strapping, it may recur and need eventual fixation with surgery. However, many players, including top county-standard goalkeepers, can play with a partially reduced acromioclavicular joint, and it does not seem to hamper them in any way. If the joint becomes painful then surgery is needed.

Fractures of the scapula are relatively unimportant because the bone heals quickly as it is surrounded by strong muscles and well protected. The only treatment is a sling for 3–4 weeks, if the shoulder is painful.

The humerus may fracture at its neck, which is in direct

relationship to the shoulder joint, and be confused with a shoulder dislocation. This fracture takes 6–12 weeks to heal and there may be some restriction of shoulder function afterwards.

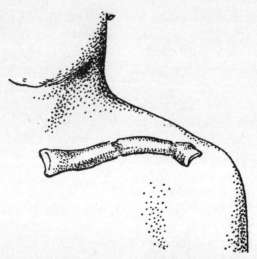

Illustration showing two common sites for fractures of the clavicle

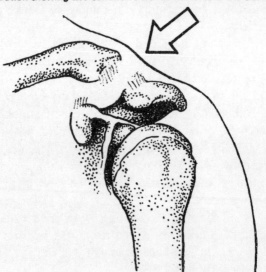

23. Fractures and dislocations of the clavicle.

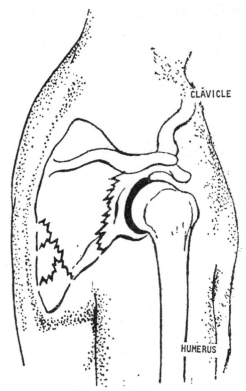

24. Fractures of the scapula.

Dislocation of the Shoulder

This injury occurs when the player falls on to an outstretched arm or shoulder so that the limb is forced outwards from the body and rotated externally. The articular head of the humerus slips out of the joint and comes to lie anteriorly, forming a prominence that can be seen and felt in front of the shoulder. At the same time the player cannot move his arm without pain, and he grasps the elbow and attempts to hold the arm in one position. Sometimes the head of the humerus passes posteriorly behind the joint. X-rays are needed to confirm the diagnosis and exclude a fracture of the humerus. Once the dislocation has

87

Football Fitness and Injuries

been reduced, a sling is worn for 2 weeks and then very gentle
mobilisation begins. If one attempts to mobilise the shoulder
before the ligaments and soft tissues have had time to heal, then
there is considerable muscle spasm and further damage may be
inflicted on the small muscles of this joint.

The final result depends upon the degree of soft tissue damage,
as mentioned in Chapter 3. If there is considerable damage the
shoulder is never fully mobile. This may not cause much difficulty in soccer players, but can affect rugger and basket-ball
players.

Some sportsmen suffer from recurrent dislocations of the
shoulder, and, depending on the amount of incapacity, surgery
may be necessary. Once again the limitation of shoulder movement imposed by surgery may affect playing performance.

*When the trainer suspects a shoulder or arm injury he should
support the limb with a well-padded sling (for shoulders) and
a collar and cuff (for the arm). The player can be transported
on a wheel-chair, which is more comfortable than a stretcher
for shoulder and arm injuries. There must be no attempt at
reduction on the field of play.*

Fractures and Dislocations in the Upper Limb

Fractures of the shaft of the humerus are uncommon in footballers, but when they occur they may be associated with radial
nerve damage, as indicated by weakness of the wrist (wrist
drop). Usually the player slips on to the hand with a straight
arm. The diagnosis is easy because there is gross swelling and
severe pain. The treatment is by a plaster U-slab or a collar-
and-cuff, for 4–8 weeks.

Fractures of the lower humeral shaft and dislocations of the
elbow will be considered together since they both present with
pain around the elbow and deformity, and what is more important, they can be complicated by artery and nerve damage.
The brachial artery runs on the front of the elbow and the
median nerve (which supplies the forearm down to the thumb)
lies close by. The radial nerve (which supplies the back of the

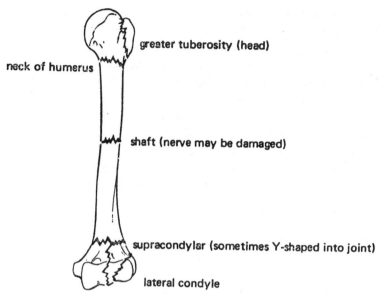

greater tuberosity (head)

neck of humerus

shaft (nerve may be damaged)

supracondylar (sometimes Y-shaped into joint)

lateral condyle

25. Fractures of the humerus.

forearm down to the tips of the fingers) and the ulnar nerve (which supplies the forearm, back and front, towards the ring and little fingers) lie respectively on the outer and inner aspect of the elbow. Any of the above four structures can be damaged with lower shaft fractures (called supracondylar fractures) and dislocations of the elbow.

Supracondylar fractures are common in children. They are caused by a fall on to a bent elbow, and the humerus breaks just above the elbow joint. The lower fragment is pushed backwards and bent inwards so that an obvious deformity is seen at the elbow. Similarly, a dislocated elbow leads to a backwards movement of the tip of the elbow (olecranon). In both injuries the radial pulse must be examined at the wrist. Medical advice is urgently needed if the pulse is absent, or if the hand develops a dusky hue.

In hospital the injury will be reduced and treated by plaster immobilisation or a collar and cuff. The player may have some permanent stiffness in the elbow joint.

The tip of the elbow can be damaged by a fall, this olecranon fracture usually needs an operation, and rest for 4–8 weeks. Although javelin throwers may tear the triceps muscle as it enters its bony attachment on the olecranon, this is a relatively uncommon injury in footballers, indicated by pain and weakness over the tip of the elbow on throwing.

The two main bones of the forearm, the radius and ulna, may be fractured individually or together. Direct blows on the forearm are the principal cause. Children develop greenstick fractures of these bones. In adults unstable fractures may need fixation with screws and plates. However, if the bones can be accurately reduced under an anaesthetic by closed methods methods (manipulation) then this injury is treated by plaster for 4–8 weeks.

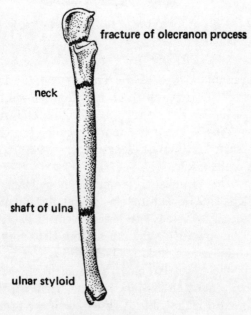

fracture of olecranon process

neck

shaft of ulna

ulnar styloid

Fractures of ulna

26. Fractures of the ulna.

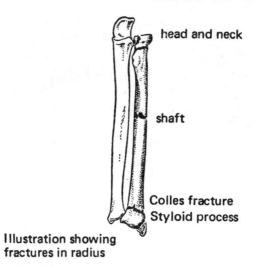

head and neck

shaft

Colles fracture
Styloid process

Illustration showing
fractures in radius

27. Fractures in the radius.

A fracture of the lower radius with backward displacement of the hand is called a Colles' fracture. This is the commonest of all fractures, more often occurring in the elderly. The classical dinner-fork deformity is seen, and pain and lack of movement at the wrist is obvious. The correct treatment is manipulation and plaster for 4–6 weeks.

All the wrist bones can be broken or dislocated, either alone or in a bewildering variety of combinations. The commonest, and most serious, is the scaphoid fracture. This is produced by a fall on to the outstretched hand, and tenderness is found on the outer aspect of the wrist. This fracture may not show on X-ray for 3 weeks, so often a plaster is applied on suspicion of scaphoid damage. Any sprain of the wrist, which is persistent, needs an X-ray to exclude the possibility of a scaphoid fracture. A plaster may have to be worn for 6–12 weeks.

Fractures of the finger bones are common in goalkeepers, the most important being the fracture of the main thumb bone (the first metacarpal) sustained when punching an awkward ball.

91

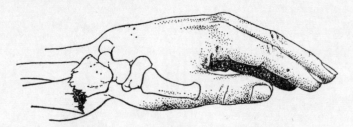

Colles fracture, showing the tilt of lower part of the radius

28. Colles fracture, showing the tilt of the lower part of the radius.

There is localised swelling at the base of the thumb with painful movements. A plaster is needed for 3–4 weeks. Fractures of the knuckles need accurate reduction and splinting to prevent deformity. The small bones of the finger are commonly dislocated, but as in all bony injuries an X-ray is of paramount importance to exclude fracture, especially into the small joints of the fingers. Despite their tiny size, any damage to the finger joints is of importance as permanent stiffness and swelling may ensue. The pernicious practice of snapping dislocated fingers back before the extent of the damage is known is to be condemned.

When the tip of the finger falls forwards due to a tear in the extensor tendon the condition is referred to as mallet finger. This injury may respond to splintage for 4–6 weeks, but can be refractory to conservative treatment. *Injuries to the elbow, forearm, wrist and hand can be supported by a padded sling, or a wood, polythene, or air splint. However, their application must not embarrass the circulation and, if in doubt, a firm sling will suffice until the limb has been seen by the club doctor.*

Fractured Ribs

A direct blow to the chest can fracture ribs, indicated by tenderness and pain on deep breathing. Fractured ribs do not need strapping, for this treatment may press the sharp ends internally, or if strapped too tightly may stop the normal respiratory excursion of the lung tissue so that stagnation and infection supervene. Ribs heal in 3 weeks, and during this period pain-killing tablets may have to be given. During the acute episode a long-acting local anaesthetic may be injected by the club doctor.

Stress fractures of the ribs are uncommon in footballers, but are sometimes found as a cause of a dull, aching chest pain.

Tears of the pectoral muscles and a localised tenderness over the costal cartilages (called the Tietz syndrome) are other causes of chest ache. All respond to a period of rest.

The importance of rib fractures lies in the fact that the sharp end of the rib may be driven internally and damage:

lung, leading to collapse and chest pain and air-hunger (pneumothorax);

liver, leading to pain and rigidity in the right side of the abdomen;

spleen, with similar symptoms and signs on the left side of the abdomen;

kidneys, leading to blood in the urine and pain in the loins.

If the trainer suspects a serious injury after a blow on the chest the player should be rested immediately and taken to Casualty.

Sometimes the lung can rupture during a game due to a congenital defect in the tissue. The onset of this spontaneous pneumothorax is heralded by chest pain, breathlessness and a thumping in the chest. I have known it come on quite suddenly in a young university rugger player while racing for touch.

Rarely, the liver, kidneys or spleen may be slightly diseased and unduly friable and thus liable to tear. For example I have witnessed a case of ruptured spleen in a young university foot-baller who was suffering from glandular fever and had an en-larged spleen as a temporary feature of the disease. This is one more reason why only fit players should participate in sporting events.

Fractures of the Pelvis

These are uncommon in footballers, and only occur after direct kicks or blows to the pelvis. The iliac crests may be cracked, and the pubic rami fractured by a blow between the legs. Pelvic injuries heal with rest for 3–6 weeks. The player may be able to walk with some difficulty, but tenderness is found along the line of the pelvic arch. Damage to the bladder, bowel and urethra may coexist with pelvic fractures, and needs medical care in hospital for several weeks. If the player receives a direct scrotal blow with diffuse tenderness of the pelvis and deep bruising, the player must not pass or attempt to pass urine until the area has been medically examined. For damage to the urethra (the outlet of the bladder) is a serious condition, and the spilling of urine into the scrotal tissues is a major complication.

When a pelvic fracture is suspected the player is covered with a blanket and carried on a firm stretcher, with the pelvis supported by sandbags or rolled blankets.

Fractures of the Lower Limb

Fractures occurring in the thigh are very serious injuries since at least two pints of blood are lost into the thigh muscles, and the patient becomes shocked. Usually a follow-through or a player falling against the thigh causes the shaft of the femur to break transversely or spirally. The sickening crack, severe pain and swelling are diagnostic.

It is unusual for a player to return to training for 6–12 months, but there are exceptions. Recovery can be hastened by nailing the femur with a K-nail.

Fractures of the lower femur can extend into the knee, and be complicated by ligament and cartilage damage which spells the end of a playing career. Any resulting knee stiffness after thigh fractures may be difficult to overcome, even after knee manipulations the player may have some permanent impairment of knee mobility.

The patella (knee-cap) can be fractured by a direct kick on to the knee or by overcontraction of the quadriceps in a sudden

FRACTURES OF THE FEMUR

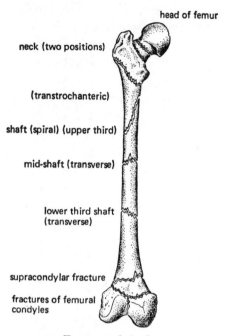

head of femur

neck (two positions)

(transtrochanteric)

shaft (spiral) (upper third)

mid-shaft (transverse)

lower third shaft
(transverse)

supracondylar fracture

fractures of femoral
condyles

29. Fractures of the femur.

unguarded movement. If the fracture is a clean break the injury
can be treated by screw or wire fixation, with plaster for 6–8
weeks. However, a comminuted fracture may need excision of
the knee cap because the resulting irregularity of the healed
fracture can irritate the knee. After patellar fractures the
quadriceps muscles will need intensive exercises, and some
permanent atrophy may be found.

The upper surface of the tibia (the tibial condyles and the
tibial spines with their cruciate and cartilage insertions) can be
fractured by direct blows or falls on the knee. Such an intra-
articular fracture causes a considerable effusion, and later stiffness in the joint. Surgery may be needed to restore the con-
tinuity of the articular surfaces. The player will need at least 6

95

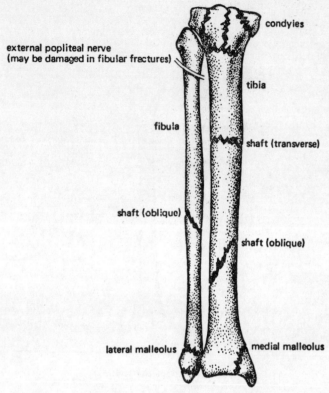

external popliteal nerve
(may be damaged in fibular fractures)

condyles

tibia

fibula

shaft (transverse)

shaft (oblique)

shaft (oblique)

lateral malleolus

medial malleolus

30. Fractures of the tibia and fibula.

weeks for partial mobilisation, but the prognosis regarding future playing is poor.

A twisting force to a stationary foot caused by a body check or a heavy tackle can fracture the tibia and fibula. Great pain ensues and the deformity and tenderness are easily seen and felt. Fractures of the tibia are one of the most common soccer fractures and it is important to recall that the muscles of the foot arise from this bone, and any subsequent weakness due to muscle atrophy by plaster immobilisation will play havoc with running, jumping and shooting.

Depending upon the nature of the tibial fracture the bone

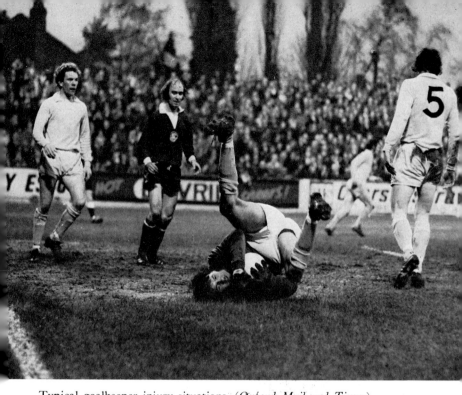

Typical goalkeeper injury situations. (*Oxford Mail and Times*)

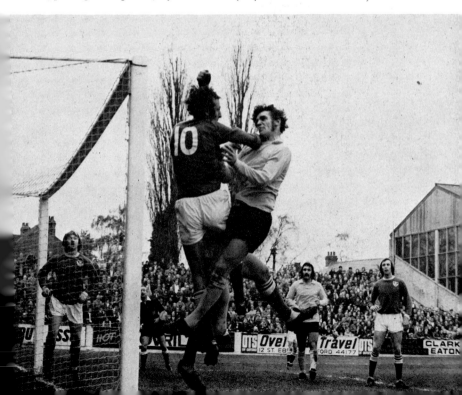

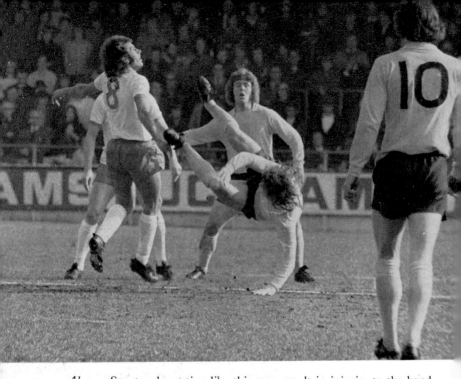

Above: Spectacular action like this may result in injuries to the hand, arm, shoulder or back. (*Oxford Mail and Times*)
Below: When players exert themselves to the maximum, injury situations can easily develop.

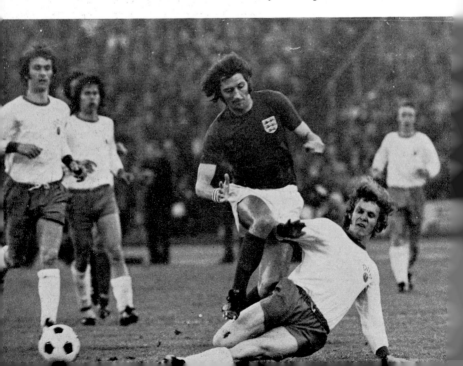

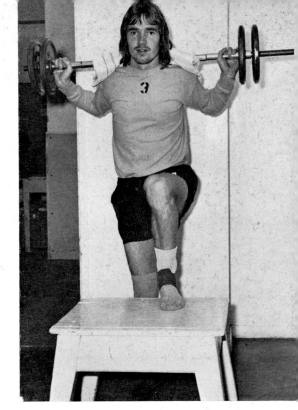

The use of weights to strengthen the muscles of the legs and back is an essential to ensure fitness. (*Jim Larkin Fotos*)

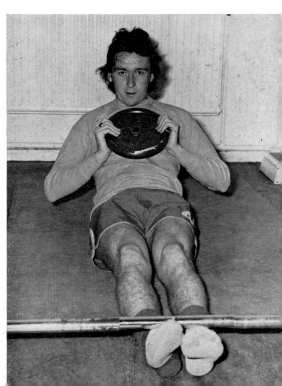

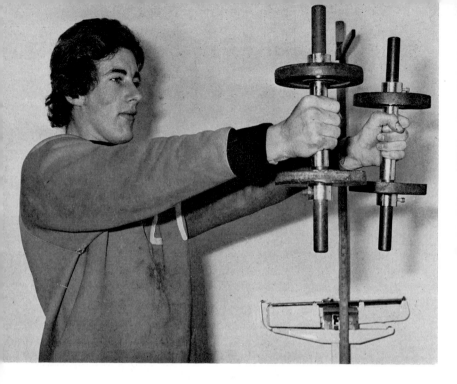

Exercises such as this with handweights help to strengthen the upper part of the body. (*Jim Larkin Fotos*)

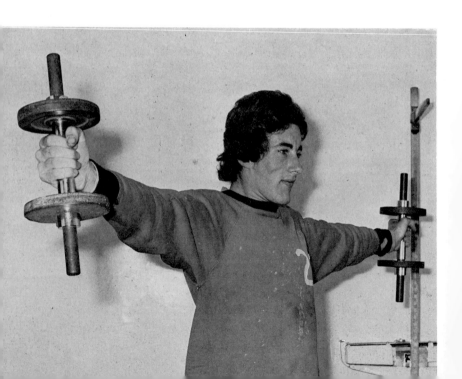

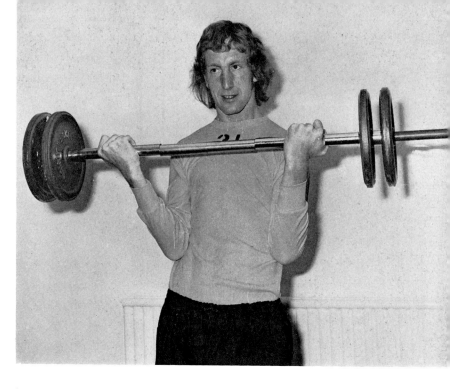

Arms and shoulders may be strengthened by using these exercises.
(*Jim Larkin Fotos*)

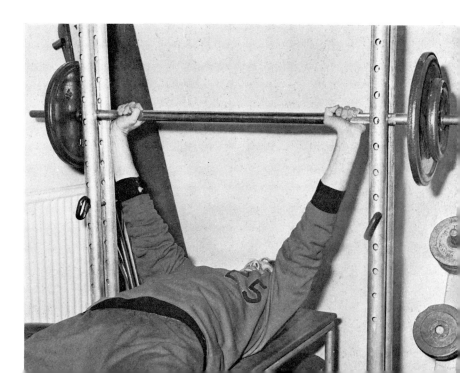

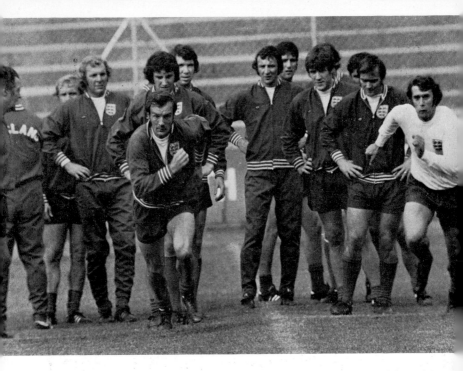

Above: The England Team in training. Speed training with sprint relays. (*Daily Mirror*)
Below: The England Team in training. Endurance is built up with a mixture of slow and fast laps. (*Daily Mirror*)

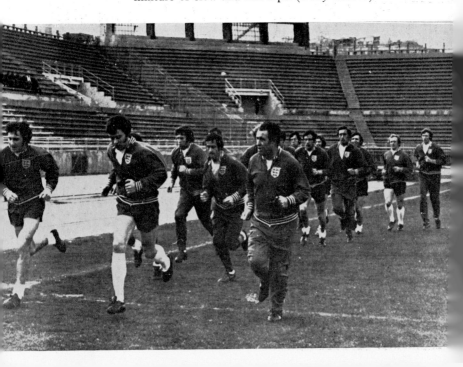

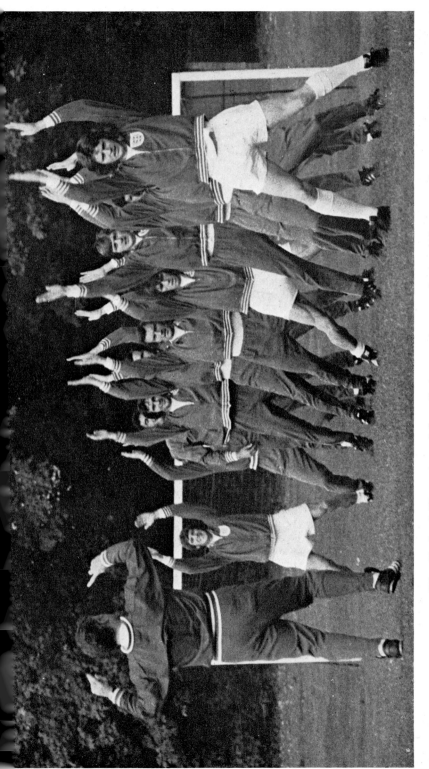

The England Team in training. Body exercises can be used for general loosening up. (*Daily Mirror*)

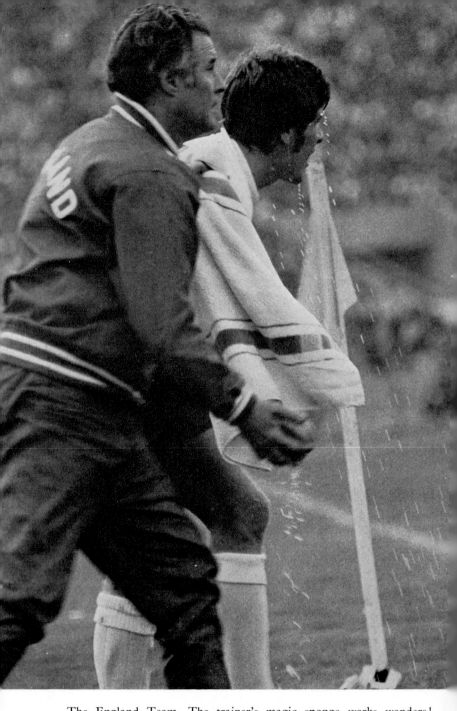

The England Team. The trainer's magic sponge works wonders!
(*Monte Fresco and Daily Mirror*)

may be treated with either plaster for 8–12 weeks; or an operation with the insertion of a bone plate may be employed. The
tibia lies just under the skin in the shin and thus the injury is
often compound which may affect the healing and prevent an
operation such as plating. On the whole, compound wounds are
a barrier to fixing a fracture with metal plates or screws.

The fibula may be fractured with the tibia, often called a
double fracture of the leg, or on its own. When the shaft of the
fibula is broken on its own the limb may not need a plaster but
only a crêpe support. Fractures of the fibula heal in 3–6 weeks.

Stress fractures may be found in the tibia or fibula and are a
cause of shin soreness. Persistent aching over a limb bone
necessitates a precautionary X-ray to exclude this simple fracture.
A reduction of training or complete rest and plaster leads to a
resolution of symptoms in 2–6 weeks.

Fractures occur in the ankle in a bewildering variety of forms,
depending on the direction of the tackle or twisting force.
Fractures of the lower end of the fibula (the lateral malleolus of
the ankle) are treated with plaster for 3–6 weeks, while fractures
of the inner aspect of the ankle (the medial malleolus) may lead
to gross instability and require surgical fixation with a screw and
plaster for 3–8 weeks (see Fig. 15).

Pott's fracture is a fracture/dislocation of the ankle which
needs accurate reduction and fixation. The true Pott's fracture
is due to a tackle directed laterally, that first of all fractures the
lateral malleolus and then tears a chip off the medial malleolus,
ultimately pushing the ankle backwards to fracture the posterior
aspect of the tibia. Gross pain and swelling accompany such an
injury. Reduction is needed under anaesthetic and a plaster is
worn for 8–12 weeks. However, surgical fixation may be needed
to accurately reduce the fragments.

The many small bones of the foot – tarsal, metatarsal and
phalanges – can be fractured alone or in combination. Fractures
of the larger bones require plaster for several weeks, but fractures of the metatarsals and phalanges may only need strapping,
although plaster immobilisation holds metatarsal fractures in a

D

snugger position. If reduction of these fractures is poorly maintained, then the resulting protuberance can cause pain and local callosities, and may require metatarsal pads or sorbo-rubber insoles.

As in upper limb injuries, leg injuries require the immediate support from crêpe and wool, or the application of a splint. The player should be carried off on a stretcher and not allowed to limp across the field, thus inflicting more damage to the muscles, ligaments and bones.

Dislocations in the Lower Limb

Dislocation of the knee is caused by severe violence, i.e. a diving tackle at rugger. Fortunately the injury is rare in soccer. However, dislocation of the patella is more common, occurring in a lateral direction. There is an obvious abnormal position of the knee cap. This dislocation can be recurrent and if so will need surgical correction.

Dislocations of the ankle are complicated by fractures of the ankle bone and the treatment is as for ankle injuries.

The small bones of the toes may be dislocated, and after reduction the player can resume training with the injury strapped in 2 weeks.

A rare injury is dislocation of the fibula head at the knee (reported in the British journal, *Sports Medicine,* in 1973). It is recognised by an abnormal lump on the outside of the patella tendon below the knee-cap. Once reduction has been achieved the player may play again in 3–6 weeks.

Miscellaneous Bony Conditions

A rare, but reported, condition in the pelvis is due to an unexplained softening of the cartilage which cements together the two halves of the pubis anteriorly. This condition is known as *osteitis pubis.* It begins as a diffuse ache in the groin region, later radiating to between the legs, and the pain is worse on standing on one leg or walking. In the early stages the pain comes on after 20 minutes or so of training, but eventually the pain is constant. An X-ray of the pelvis reveals tilting of the pelvis and softening of the pubic bones at their junction. The condition usually remits spontaneously in 2–3 months (as in the cases of Alan Mullery, Bob McNab and Hugh Curran), but during this period strict rest is required initially (2–3 weeks) and then light graduated exercises. Anti-inflammatory tablets can help, but short-wave diathermy, manipulations and ultrasound are not usually effective. Refractory cases may need a bone graft across the pubis.

A dull aching pain in the region of the heel on the sole of the foot can be due to a strain of the ligaments (called *plantar fasciitis*). It is much more common in long jumpers and hurdlers. Although an X-ray of the heel may show an additional spike of bone, this condition usually responds to hydrocortisone injections and a sorbo-rubber pad in the boot.

Although this chapter has described a large number of fractures, luckily such injuries are uncommon in footballers, and of those that do occur, most are minor in nature.

Chapter Six

Fitness, Nutrition and Health

It goes without saying that all three topics are interdependent, and an understanding of one requires a basic consideration of another. But fitness and health are abstract phenomena which often defy simple descriptions.

Each sporting activity makes a general demand on the cardiovascular system, muscles, joints, etc., but every sport also makes specific demands on certain organs or structures, e.g. the enormous increase in arm muscles in a tennis star, the powerful quadriceps of the soccer player.

But the old saying that 'athletes are born not made' has a general ring of truth about it.

A study of physical forms has produced the following classification:

endomorph, described as a roundness of physique and a capacity to store fat, the Oliver Hardys of this world;

mesomorph, seen as the Tarzan muscular group;

ectomorph, means a slimness of build, the Stan Laurels of the populace.

However, very few people conform to this absolute rule, and there are slight variations around the theme. The typical endomorph is usually genial and expansive; the ectomorph is in direct contrast to the endomorph – quiet, shy, retiring;

while the mesomorph is often aggressive, thriving on competition.

I mention these fundamental aspects of human form because although I am conscious of their 'general nature', it behoves the trainer or coach to view the athlete as a whole, observing not just the physical form but the mental make-up behind it. Many players look the part, but lack fire. Others are awkward, and look as if they have been composed of heavenly remnants, but their drive and determination make them match-winners. It is amazing how a team, certainties on paper, fails to rise to the occasion; whereas one or two seemingly innocuous ansertions can transform the team spirit by their very competitive fature.

A study of Olympic athletes has shown that swimmers and wrestlers have a high fat component (a tendancy to endomorph structure), while the addition of androgenic steroids (illegal) to the menu have distorted the outline of the throwers of discus, hammer and shot towards frank endomorphy. However, the mesomorphic power of the sprinter and long jumper is easily recognisable, while the need for longer legs and lighter body weight by the distance runner places him in the reticent, ectomorph class.

No amount of weight-training or running will convert one distinct body form to another. But the player can be directed by a shrewd trainer into the sport to which he is best suited. Luckily, most budding soccer stars have become proficient in one position before they embark on higher grades, and this is partly reached under the natural competition boys have on the playing fields, or school grounds.

But the trainer or manager will often have to depend for future success on the development of a youth policy without really being able to spot the winners. Some players ripen at an early age, and their very ability is obvious as early as 16 years (Denis Law is an excellent example) while others have all the physical attributes and skill yet seem to languish in the backwaters without being spotted for several years (Rodney Marsh and Hugh Curran both had several clubs before their outstanding ability was spotted).

So what are the questions a trainer must ask himself about the young apprentice? And how long should he ask them?

A good trainer or coach will have a player under some form of surveillance from 12 to 21 years. The success of many youth policies, e.g. at Manchester United and Burnley, has tempted most clubs to spend a great deal of time and money on players in the 15–18 age bracket, It is not generally realised that in some players both maturity in muscle and bones may be delayed to 19–21 years, and that an 18-year-old discard is a possible star of tomorrow. After all, Len Shackleton was an Arsenal cast-off. It should also be apparent to most trainers that although strength will increase with age, speed will diminish. Thus a player who is too slow at 15 years, will only marginally improve in swiftness as the years go by, and no amount of weight-training will make a slow runner a sprinter. However, endurance – which is dependant on heart and lung reserves – can be improved with training. Finally, the most genetically endowed factor is skill, which must be present from the beginning. A basic, innate skill with a ball can be brought out, fostered and matured by good training and coaching. It should be possible to assess any skill potential in 1–2 weeks, and if present the player should improve in 1–2 months. Players who reach a plateau after only a short period (4–8 weeks) of intensive training, usually are a dead loss from the playing point of view. Similarly, if a young player has all the basic ingredients of soccer stardom, he must have drive and determination. It is always wise to assess the psychological aspect of each one individually. Some players respond to criticism or 'bullying'; others do not, and become more withdrawn.

In summary a good player needs:

strength, depending on his body configuration; this can be increased with age and training;

skill, dependant on complex nervous and muscular pathways; partly inborn, and partly acquired;

speed, almost wholly inborn; depending upon the number of fast moving muscle fibres, the arrangement of bony structures and nerve reflexes;

endurance, has its basis in good general health and nutrition; can be increased by good heart and lung exercises, by repetitive running;

drive and determination, may be inborn or acquired, can be encouraged by the correct psychological approach, but limited by a player's personality (see also Chapter 8). Some players lack the necessary drive and ambition to be successful, either on the field of play, or as self-discipline during training.

Training aims at building up the cardio-vascular and respiratory reserves by a combination of short sprints admixed with longer running, jogging and walking; with an increase in the more severe exercises as the standard of fitness improves. Weight training can then be utilised to increase muscle mass (i.e. the 'red' fibres, connective and vascular tissues) and at the same time it takes the joints through a full range of movement, thus improving the extensibility of tendons and ligaments necessary for peak performance.

It would be presumptious to detail all training methods in a book on injuries but certain basic facts must be observed (see also Chapter 8).

The key to successful training is variety. Some trainers persevere with the same old routine to the boredom and unmitigated annoyance of the players. A good coach sits down and thinks 'What activities are mundane?', and he does something about it. A country trip in a variety of surroundings adds interest compared to lapping the perimeter of the pitch. Competitions, by splitting up the team into small groups, heightens enjoyment especially if rewards like a game of squash or golf are given to the winning group. Ball games are always fun, and although amongst ball-players stress should always be laid on their sport (in this case football), other ball games will give added diversion and training at the same time.

Do not injure the player during training. There is nothing more annoying to a club doctor than dealing with training injuries. Players have a great capacity for striking each other with golf balls, squash raquets and unusual parts of their antomy. Players should also be protected from hard floors, uneven or rutted pitches and heavy conditions during training especially if there is a history of chronic ankle or knee trouble. Obviously during poor wintry weather there are times when indoor training is a must, but the trainer must use his judgement in the duration of playing, the type of exercises and the nature of the footwear.

Always be aware of the signs of overtraining. Never allow athletes to strain under gigantic loads in so-called weight training. Select the maximum comfortable lift for each area concerned and reduce it by 20 lb. or so. Then use this weight for repeated exercises. Do not carry out a manoeuvre with the weights until a dull pain or aching is felt. These symptoms indicate minor damage to the structures. Straining under heavy weights is useless, and eventually permanent damage can be inflicted on ligaments and joints.

Have base lines on performance for each player. Every player is an individual in his own right, and proficiency in one form of training may mean that he can spend his valuable time on other aspects at which he is not so good, e.g. an excellent sprinter does not need repeated bursts up and down the track. He may need jumping or heading practice. To see players wasting their time on exercises that they can do backwards is an affront to their ability, and extremely boring! But this fact emerges only too often if one questions players closely. If the trainer knows the performance of each player and has a record accurately charted, he can compare performance at weekly intervals and determine the amount of training on the particular facet that player needs. Coaches do not realise the relatively small amount of training which can maintain performance, for example only 5 minutes of muscular exercise a day can maintain muscle bulk, and repeated short bursts of activity are much better than long, single efforts.

Do not allow players to train before fully fit. After an injury all ranges of movement, active and passive, should be tested. There are lots of simple tests to stress once-injured limbs, e.g. press-ups for the arms, crouch-springing for the calves, and the trainer and coach should become familiar with a few and use them in a standard fashion. Thus a graph or recovery chart can be made on each injured player, and the eventual return to fitness exactly determined.

But the golden rule remains – never rush a player back to training – and accept a slow return to full activity. Be patient with players, encourage and show an interest in their problems. Be frank, and if you think there are superadded personal or psychological problems, sort them out as well.

Nutrition and Sport

Nutrition in sportsmen is bedevilled with superstition and faddism, hence the pressure on sportsmen from the advertising media to take this, swallow that and drink the other for extra strength. One fact emerges from these curious food practices: athletes have little or no idea what happens to the food they ingest, and most of their theories are based on historical precedents. For example, one of the most popular diets in training and before a match has been based on a high protein diet, consumed as large quantities of meat, supposedly destined to replace the protein lost during muscular activity. The Greeks had employed a vegetarian diet supplemented with a little meat during athletic events, but after Roman times more and more meat was eaten, especially by the boxers and wrestlers, and a high protein diet became equated with great strength. Many more bizarre nutritional beliefs echo Roman thought and medieval superstition. Honey, wheat-germ, raw meat, plant extracts have all had their vogue in sport, but at the end of the day the conclusion can be made: *the recommended diet for sportsmen is no different than that suggested for a normal person, except in the need for more calories.*

Each healthy person requires carbohydrates, fats and protein in a balanced proportion, with a very small amount of vitamins and minerals. The proportions of each constituent are: carbohydrates 4, fats 1, protein 1. The normal daily requirement for an average worker is 2,500–3,000 calories; whereas a footballer may need almost double this amount.

Dishes with a high protein intake seem to be the preferred choice of sportsmen, although the ingestion of protein does not stimulate human muscle growth or increase performance. However, the position with regard to fats and carbohydrates is quite different, because these substances provide the energy for working muscles; and once the energy source becomes depleted then muscle performance falls and activity stops. The relative amount of fat and carbohydrate determines the percentage of each burnt during exercise. Given a 24-hour delay (on average) carbohydrates and fats, and some proteins, can be stored in the muscle fibre as glycogen (animal starch composed of many units of glucose). Glycogen (as glucose) is the high-octane fuel of exercise, and for that extra burst to win a match the players must not run out of glycogen before the final whistle.

Unfortunately many players do burn up their energy long before the end of the match, and this is seen as sluggish recovery, poor skill especially ball distribution, cramps, incoordination and increased proneness to over-use injuries.

Thus the glycogen content of working muscle is one of the most important factors for continued prolonged exercise. It has been shown that exercise to exhaustion can reduce muscle glycogen to almost zero, but it can be built up to almost four times the normal level by a high carbohydrate diet.

Let us suppose that the big match or event is on a Saturday. What happens in club 'A'?

Trainer Dim takes his team out for a heavy exercise programme on Friday, including a 3-mile run, a few short, sharp bursts in heavy mud and shooting practice on a bumpy practice pitch with old, irregular balls. On Saturday he races the players round for 30 minutes, keeps them anxious by barking incoherent orders all morning, then allows them a miniscule piece of fish for the meal before the match.

Trainer Smart meanwhile has worked his players to exhaustion on Thursday, and on Friday has given them light limbering exercises. He has encouraged them to take a high carbohydrate diet (cereals, sweets, liquid glucose, sugars, bread, etc.) and allowed time for the glycogen stores to be rebuilt on the Friday afternoon and Saturday morning. On the match day he keeps the players relaxed so that they are not burning-up nervous energy (like a car with the choke out) and gives them a high carbohydrate breakfast and lunch (the latter is suplemented by liquid glucose). Thus club 'B' has prepared with forethought and intelligence.

The result is a sweeping victory for club 'B'.

The following graphs show the effect of such a dietary regimen supplemented by liquid glucose. It is quite apparent that team performance as assessed by goals for and against, ball contact and participation are all improved after the special training regimen (ref: *British Journal of Sports Medicine* page 340, 1973).

In the prisoners who tottered out of concentration camps in the last war there was frank evidence of vitamin deficiency, and their whole muscular co-ordination was impaired. However, on a normal average diet there is never any vitamin deficiency for the amount of these substance required daily is very, very small. Thus clubs only waste their money by providing vast loading doses of vitamins, and some (like vitamins A and D) can be toxic in excess amounts and detrimental to health. This fact is not appreciated by the layman. For example vitamin C, being water-soluble, is simply passed through the kidneys once a certain level has been reached, and even if a player was depleted of all vitamin C for several weeks his body level would only fall slightly because of the reserves in the tissues. No club doctor

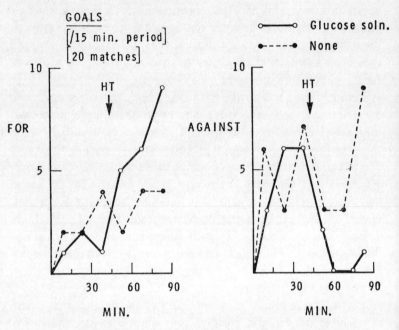

31. Goals – for and against after liquid glucose regimen.

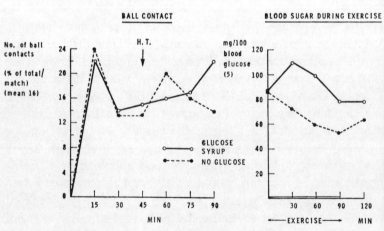

32. Ball contact and blood sugar estimations after liquid glucose regimen.

	NO GLUCOSE		GLUCOSE SYRUP	
	1st. half	2nd. half	1st. half	2nd. half
F	8	10 (8)	4	20 (15)
A	16	15 (12)	15	3 (1)

Figures in brackets indicate goals in last 30 mins of match
33. Goals in last 30 minutes – non-glucose and glucose.

SCORING EFFORTS

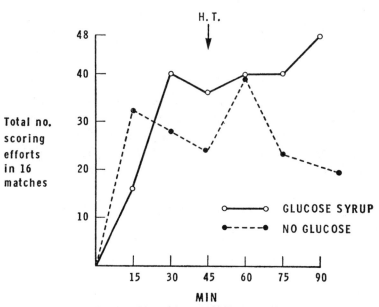

34. Scoring efforts after liquid glucose regimen.

objects to the occasional administration of vitamins and tonics, but their excessive use is to be deprecated.

The importance of mineral intake is obvious when one recalls the fact that sodium and chloride is lost during sweating. There are many salt solutions on the market which can be given after exercise to replace salt loss. However, most players obtain sufficient minerals from a normal healthy diet. It has been reported that professional athletes can destroy red blood corpuscles during exercise and thus become iron deficient. There is a good case for testing the haemoglobin level in all players at the beginning of each season, but at Oxford only one player was found to be slightly anaemic. He responded to iron tablets.

General Health

The general health of sportsman must be good to give peak performance. It is also a fact that a simple illness like influenza can take 2–3 weeks to get over, and performance may be slightly down during this recovery period. Once the body is invaded by germs, certain changes occur in the tissue cells, and their outline becomes swollen and their interior cloudy in appearance. All cells of the liver, kidney, heart, muscles, etc. suffer this change, and this alteration gives rise to a feeling of malaise and general ill health. Until these changes revert back to normal the athlete functions below par. Thus every infection should be treated seriously from the beginning, and the player given bed rest, appropriate medication and a good diet. They should be discouraged from wandering round in thin, open-shirts, coughing all over colleagues, drinking from the same utensils, sitting in cold draughty rooms, and hanging around coffee bars and fish-and-chip shops.

A club can lose more playing time from minor infections than from injuries. This is especially so during winter when colds and 'flu' are rife. The use of influenza vaccines has been disappointing unless the strain of virus has been identified in a serious outbreak. The trainer should seek medical advice on this matter early in the season, because it is no use waiting until half the club is ill with 'flu' before obtaining the vaccine. Tonsillitis is also commonly due to a virus (about 60 per cent of cases) and this makes the use of antibiotics such as penicillin and tetracycline debatable. However, since about 40 per cent of sore throats can be cured with antibiotics, and in other cases secondary infection impeded by these drugs, club doctors usually advise their administration in this disease.

Gastro-enteritis outbreaks usually settle in 2–6 days, and in many instances the organisms which cause mild food poisoning are not often sensitive to medication. Fluid loss (as graphically depicted in Chapter 7) can be a serious problem and the player must be well hydrated. Antibiotics such as the sulphonamide derivatives, 'Penbritin,' neomycin, etc., are given in serious cases.

Fungal infections are common in footballers and are picked up in communal baths and showers. These germs cause trouble, especially when they irritate the groins (causing a diffuse, circular, itching red area) and between the toes (causing peeling of skin, weeping, and offensive smell). The broken skin between the toes allows other more serious bacteria to enter the skin and cause a spreading cellulitis.

In the World Cup of 1966, and subsequently, every minute detail which might have any bearing on the players' physical and mental attitude to their task was given the strictest attention, and this included the care of the toe-nails and feet. It might seem inappropriate for professional footballers to need instruction on the care of their feet. Yet at the daily foot inspections there was a demonstration on how to cut toe-nails, with details of how the smallest of sharp points from an incorrectly cut toe-nail could lead to a skin puncture, which might cause infection and jeopardise a player's fitness and could also affect the balance of the modern lightly built cut-away football boot.

Fungal infections of the toes (athlete's foot) need rigorous daily cleansing with a mild antiseptic, and the application of an antifungal cream or powder (such as 'Mycil' or 'Jadit'). Most of the team will require treatment at once to eradicate the fungus, and the baths and showers need cleaning with a strong antiseptic.

Finally, in the topic of infections, the recent upsurge in venereal disease amongst young persons has caught up with the athletic fraternity. The presence of an urethral discharge – usually purulent and in the morning specimen of urine – associated with itching, redness and a painless (sometimes painful) penile spot or lump, requires urgent medical advice. There is no need to emphasise the dangers of non-treatment, which are possible insanity and death. Penicillin and related antibiotics will kill off the infection .

The conscientious trainer is always alert to the maintenance of good general health of his players apart from injuries (which take up most of his time). He is also required to keep an eye on the food before matches, know the hotel for comfort, warmth and cooking, see that his players get a good night's rest (free from personal anxieties), pander to their occasional food whims and, in all, act as overlord to the party.

Despite meticulous preparation in every respect, the occasional mishap still occurs. In the first match of the 1966 World Cup (England *v.* Uruguay) the pre-match calm was shattered by the revelation that seven of the English players were not eligible for the game because they had forgotten the little red passports, which established their identity, as demanded by the FIFA. These identity cards had to be handed to the referee before the kick-off. So the months of planning, the years of waiting, and the interest and excitement of a 100,000 Wembley crowd and millions of television, depended upon the rapid return of these little red books. To add to the confusion the players, in their pre-match tension, had forgotten where they had put the documents ... 'In my blue suit' ... 'In the top right-hand dressing-table' ... vaguely ... 'In my passport, I think ... unless its with my shirts.' A police motor cyclist raced off to the hotel, and after a frantic search by the staff, and a hair-raising journey back on the wrong side of the road most of the way, sometimes on the pavement when the whole of the road had been given over to one way traffic, the precious identity cards were retrieved, with only forty minutes to spare! Even in the midst of the worry, Jack Charlton mumbled: 'Man, they don't need identity cards at Leeds... everybody knows me up there!'

Such are the responsibilities of the trainer – away from the treatment room.

Chapter Seven

The Magic Sponge

Although the standard work of the average trainer is the treatment of soft tissue injuries, either when they happen or the necessary remedial exercises later, the trainer's responsibilities extend much farther than this simple concept. Not only is he the qualified expert in the needs of the footballer, he is their sympathetic adviser as well.

So when asked what are the essential qualities required in a good trainer, one would confidently suggest a quiet, but knowledgeable person, with an easily approachable personality. Because the trainer has to spend many hours with a player after injury, teaching him therapeutic exercises, and during this period there must develop a close bond of respect. The trainer will be asked questions way beyond those concerned with the injury; social, domestic, financial and emotional problems will be discussed. Often it is the trainer who first finds the seeds of discontent which may lead to a transfer request later; and, in the case of very serious injuries, the player will draw on the trainer's knowledge of other players who have sustained similar troubles and whether they ever returned to the game. Also, simple worries away from the ground can affect players, especially the young apprentices and ground staff. It may be a question of poor lodgings and food, or suppressed homesickness. Because of the latter Eric McMordie left Manchester United, having gone there with George Best, and returned to Ireland. He later agreed to sign for Middlesbrough and won an international cap.

However, the majority of trainers are not concerned with £100,000 plus players, apprentice accommodation, good hotels and transport, vaccinations and scouting. The greatest number of trainers are those concerned with the thousands of small clubs at village, works or school level. These men have as much responsibility as the professional trainer, for the average club player is entirely in the hands of these part-time trainers, medical advice is not immediately available except in the case of major injuries, and the player may limp around all week-end with a minor bruise or strains before going to the local general practitioner on a Monday morning. Since many future stars pass through his ambit, the amateur trainer must have a working knowledge of the principles of anatomy, first aid, soft tissue injuries and their immediate treatment, and the possible complications of both injury and inadequate therapy. It is not a job to be taken lightly, and yet it combines a fascinating mixture of medicine, sport and exercise. However, being the trainer of a football club means more than running out on to the pitch with a wet sponge, or applying a crêpe bandage to a swollen knee. The normal bumps and bruises of soccer demand instant treatment, and this regimen includes an accurate diagnosis on the field of play, be it Wembley Stadium or the local park. It is not enough to apply the magic sponge, ease pain and then allow the player to rush back into activity. Often the circumstance of the injury (a collision of heads or a high-tackle) may give a ready clue to the trainer as to the type of damage sustained, while the degree of injury can only be assessed as the initial examination is being carried out on the pitch – or perhaps not even then, where there are complications. Since some players over-react, a sound insight into their characters and response to pain must be obtained.

The knowledge that any injury will be treated promptly, diligently and correctly can only give added confidence to the players, and this is reflected in individual and team performance.

In this respect both the manager and trainer have an important part to play. The sensational success of Ipswich in winning the First Division Championship, and England in the 1966 World Cup, must be attributable to the confidence the players had in the manager, Sir Alf Ramsey and his organisation, for he was always diligent in avoiding the chance of causing unrest and insecurity amongst the players by unfair criticism, and if any player was dropped he was always at pains to tell him the reason for the decision. He made it clear that players would not be dropped on the evidence of one indifferent performance.

The great team spirit in the England side was manifestly evident in the World Cup final at Wembley in 1966. Helmut Schoen had said, 'To be second in this match will be no disgrace,' and with only moments remaining the German Team Manager's words seemed to be coming true. However, with only about fifteen seconds left, Weber stretched out a long right foot and hooked the ball under the diving Gordon Banks. The excitement amongst the 100,000 crowd was intense, and it radiated out via television to over 400,000,000 people around the world. To recover from such a shattering psychological blow was perhaps one of England's greatest achievements. While all of us tried to massage new vigour into tired and aching muscles, Sir Alf Ramsey simply told his men: 'You have won it once. Now go out and win it again.' Geoff Hurst's goals put the issue beyond doubt. It was a triumph of teamwork, meticulous planning and attention to detail both on and off the field.

When travelling around as Trainer to the England Team one was always aware of the responsibility of the job. In England we have no problems in the treatment of injuries, for any medical requisite is readily available and expert surgical or medical treatment only a telephone call away. Playing abroad is a different proposition, especially in some Eastern European countries where it is often not easy to get hold of the type of commodity you specifically require. Therefore, whenever an England team goes on tour, I endeavour to take with me sufficient medical supplies to cover the whole trip, whether it be one game or six. It is important to be a self-contained unit and I try to visualise our needs for the trip. Apart from the treatment of sprains, cuts and bruises, the further treatment and rehabilitation of injuries goes on. For this purpose a couple of infra-red lamps are always carried in the kit.

I was first appointed as England Trainer in 1957 and in those days a doctor never accompanied the team on any occasion. This omission, of course, placed a terrible responsibility on my shoulders. Whilst I was capable of dealing with the normal, run-of-the-mill football injury, it was absolutely essential that a doctor should be a member of the party for obvious reasons.

The practice used to be that if a doctor was needed we called upon the hosts to provide one. This never proved to be a satisfactory arrangement. There was always the language barrier, the players naturally lacked confidence in the foreigner administering the treatment, and time was involved. Two experiences readily spring to mind.

In 1960, when England were touring Hungary, Bobby Robson went down with tonsillitis. We were staying at Lake Balaton some 100 miles out of Budapest. After confining Bobby to bed for a day, I suggested to Walter Winterbottom, our team manager, that he ought to have some penicillin injections. So we managed to obtain a local doctor – a charming man, obviously overworked and underpaid, and with only a few words of English at his command – to help him with his diagnosis.

The doctor agreed (through an interpreter) that Bobby needed penicillin, but in Hungary at this time the drug was in very short supply. To the doctor's credit he managed to produce sufficient to administer to the player's needs. However, because he was so busy he was only able to visit every two days, so in fact the player was treated intermittently and kept out of action for almost twice as long as he should have been.

To add to our troubles, the next day Johnny Haynes got a fish bone lodged in his throat and had to be taken 100 miles into Budapest to see another doctor before the offending bone could be removed.

Another alarming experience occurred in the 1962 World Cup finals in Chile.

Peter Swan contracted a very serious attack of gastro-enteritis. Again we were out in the wilds, our training camp being some 3,500 feet up on the slopes of the Andes, at a copper mine. I took the normal precautions of isolating the player, confining him to bed, keeping him on fluids and administering tablets that could have settled the infection. However, Peter showed no response and his condition deteriorated. It became obvious that medical advice was imperative. We managed to obtain the help of a local doctor, who despite the language barrier, didn't seem unduly perturbed. He gave the patient some medicine and stated that it would clear up the infection. To cut a long story short – Peter's condition deteriorated even more, and because of fluid loss he developed dehydration. The situation was such that the player needed hospitalisation. This is what actually happened: Walter Winterbottom called in the local World Cup representative and arrangements were made for the player's transfer to a hospital in Santiago. We later received a message that Swan's condition had improved, but that the transfer was none too early. Here again five valuable days were lost!

However, in 1963 the situation completely changed. When Sir Alf Ramsey was appointed as Team Manager, one of his first appointments was Dr Alan Bass, Medical Officer to Arsenal, as Englands' Team Doctor. From there, further appointments were made ensuring that every England Team – be it senior, under 23, youth or amateur – had its own doctor. Now there is a thorough organisation to swing into action every time an International match is played, either in Great Britain, or abroad. Dr Neil Phillips, the present England Medico, has at his disposal the best that medical services can offer, should the need arise. Orthopaedic surgeons are available for urgent consultation, and if any international player is seriously hurt at Wembley, it is only a matter of a very short time before he is receiving the best medical attention it is possible to obtain.

Similarly, when we are abroad the doctor makes contact with

local hospitals and specialists to arrange medical facilities should
an injury occur. A classical example of the thoroughness of Dr
Phillips arrangements was seen in Mexico during the 1970
World Cup. With all due respect to the Mexicans and their
hospital services, it was felt that if we had any serious injury
such as a fracture, the best possible treatment could be obtained
at Houston in Texas – a matter of 1 hour's flying time from
Guadalajara. So the British Ambassador made available an aero-
plane to stand by should any player require hospital treatment.
So, every time England took the field in Mexico, a plane stood
ready on the tarmac ready to fly to Houston at a moment's
notice.

The normal run of injuries in the England squad can be dealt
with quite capably within the organisation of doctor and trainer
working in close harmony. Obviously the players have more
confidence in someone they have accepted as part of the team.
During our preparation for matches, Dr Phillips is with the team
the whole of the time and any eventuality is well catered for. I
often shudder when I think of those early days, especially when
one evaluates the merchandise involved. In turn, it is only fair
to the clubs to see that their players are correctly cared for
while with the England team.

The elaborate facilities of the International team are not
available in such magnitude to the average soccer club, and at
the lowest rung of the football ladder, the only person who is
asked to deal with an injury situation is the referee.

When a player is injured the most important thing to remember, as in all First Aid, is to use common sense. Although there
are many slight bumps which recover with the application of the
magic sponge, my own theory over the years, as I run on the
field to attend to an injured player, is to expect the worst and
hope for the best. In these days of substitutes always advise the
injured player to leave the field if in doubt as to the seriousness
of the injury. Once in the dressing room the necessary therapy
can be given coolly and deliberately, away from the haste of the
playing pitch.

All clubs should have a first aid kit, organised by the trainer or club doctor. I think referees could spell out a gospel here by asking teams to provide reasonable medical kits with sterile lint dressings. The club does not need unlimited stocks of materials, but it is a disgrace to see a player in a minor club led off the field by someone clutching a dirty towel or sponge over a nasty cut. An adequate first aid kit is not very expensive and is in the interest of the players! The following kit is what I suggest for the average club trainer. Remember, it must be replenished regularly. There is no point in having an empty tin around the place. It gives false confidence!

Trainer's Medical Requirements for Senior Team

Cotton Wool $\frac{1}{2}$ lb. pkts.(2)

Absorbent Gauze

Elastic Adhesive Bandages 3 in. (2 doz.)

First Aid Strip 3 in. (6 pkts)

White Zinc Oxide Plasters 1 in. (6)

Lint Dressings (6)

Penicillin Tulle (2)

Chiropody Felt

Cotton Bandages 2 in. (2 doz.) and 3 in. (2 doz.)

Conforming Bandages 3 in. (1 doz.)

Tubigrip (Knee and Ankle)

Crêpe Bandages 3 in. (6), 2 in. (6) and 6 in. (6)

Triangular Bandages (2)

Adhesive Sponge Rubber (1 box)

Elastic Knee Bandages (2)

Elastic Anklets (2)

Sterile Gauze Pads (6)

Sterispon (1 roll)

Pneumatic Readi-Splints (2 – leg and arm)

Skefron Sprays (2)

Chiropody Kit with Disposable Scalpels (1)

Nobecutane Spray (50 gr.)

Mycil Powder and Ointment (50 gr.)

Surgical Spirit (250 ml.)

Cicatrin Powder (30 gr.)

Cetavlex Cream (2 tubes)

Betnovate Cream (1 tube)

Chloromycetin Cream and Eye Ointment (15 gr.)

Otrivine Spray (1)

Vick (2 jars)

Dextrosol Tablets (3 pkts.) or Liquid Glucose

Smelling Bottles (2)

Desogen Tablets (6 pkts.)

Panadol Tablets (1 bottle)

Olive Oil

Scissors (4 pairs)	Sterile Eye Wash
Embrocation (2 bottles)	Clinical Thermometer
Vaseline (4 jars)	Talcum Powder (3 tins)
Algipan (4 tubes)	Shampoos (20)
Xylocaine Ointment 1%	Chewing Gum (20)
(2 tubes)	

I have experienced so much difficulty in obtaining a bucket whilst on tour that in desperation I used to take my own with me. I purchased an ordinary camper's bucket and made sure when the kit was being packed that this valuable piece of equipment went in the kitbag first. The sponge is, of course, the simplest way of transporting a volume of water and the shock effect of cold water being doused over a player may be quite magical (as the title of this chapter implies). I have received many letters throughout the years from people who thought that some weird and wonderful potion was in the sponge bag. One person wrote back to me and said he didn't believe that it was only cold water and inferred that I was loathe to give away a trainer's well-guarded secret.

Cold water came in handy in the World Cup in England (especially against Argentine, when the temperature was in the 80s and Rattin's slow exit from the field after being sent off, gave me time to give our boys a welcome cool off) and in Mexico. But the sponge can be used to apply cold or hot compresses to bruised thighs, knees and ankles (cold in the early stages, warm when the injury has settled down). So don't forget the handy bucket and sponge!

Additional Medical Requirements for the Club Doctor

These include:

A stretcher, splints, wooden board or support for spinal injuries.

A supply of varying sizes of crêpe and cotton bandages, including a triangular bandage.

Sterile dressings of various sizes, cotton-wool, tulle gras, elasto-plast and other adhesive plasters.

Adhesive felt padding.

Mild antiseptic solutions like Dettol, T.C.P., Hibitane etc.

A supply of warm water, and cold ice cubes (plus towel, hot-water bottle or polythene bag. A proprietary brand of cooling solution can be used).

Adrenaline solution for nose bleeds.

Eye bath.

Dumb-bell sutures.

Black silk sutures, catgut, nylon suture, dexon, needles, forceps, scissors and local anaesthetic.

Syringes and needles of various sizes.

Steroids for injection.

Local anaesthetic spray.

Aspirins, Indomethacin, Butazolidin, Ibuprofen analgesics. Antacids. Anti-diarrhoeal pills and medicine. Sleeping pills. Antibiotics (Penicillin V, Penbritin, Cloxacillin, Tetracycline).

Antibiotic skin sprays, local 'plastic' covering sprays for abrasions.

Oral dispersing agents (e.g. Ananase, Chymoral etc.).

Tetanus toxoid.

Other medications can be ordered at the discretion of the doctor.

Chapter Eight

Team Training

The attainment and maintenance of muscle power depends upon a correct training in progressive exercises which gradually prepare the footballer for vigorous exertion, and help him to achieve his best performance.

Before starting an activity most sportsmen 'warm up'. It is still not clear whether this period, which can vary from 10 to 30 minutes, actually improves performance, but there is no doubt that it has great benefit in preventing pulled muscles and also in allaying anxiety before an event. Most pulled muscles act over two joints in an antagonistic manner, e.g. the hamstrings extend the hip but flex the knee. Uncoordinated contraction tears muscle fibres, and antagonists must relax while prime movers contract. Thus to obtain a good muscle stretch the limbs must be moved slowly and not in a jerky manner. However, it is quite common to see jerky movements being employed, such as hasty toe-touching exercises or vigorous trunk bending.

As a preliminary to the main training programme a carefully thought-out warming-up session is the ideal preparation for the player, both physically and psychologically. Over the past few decades much has been said, and many experiments and a great deal of scientific investigation have taken place (particularly in the United States) into the value of the warming-up period for athletes, whether before an event or before a training session. Arguments both for and against warm-ups have been propounded and, as often appears to be the case with subjects relating to the technical side of coaching and training, soccer in the main has cocked an ear to these debates, and has dabbled in the results of all the research and conjecture, but until very recently systematic programmes of training (of which the warm-up is an integral component) have been conspicuous throughout British football by their absence!

Progressive Training

The balance is now beginning to tip the other way, but, even so, there may be numerous professional clubs whose training schedules are not planned or geared to the specific needs of the player in relation to the tasks he is asked to perform and the physical ability required to carry out such tasks.

All training programmes should be progressive, and this applies particularly to football. A sound training programme must be arranged in accordance with the capabilities of the players for whom it is intended and in relation to the work they undertake. The programme must gradually increase in difficulty or severity from session to session, so as to ensure steady and systematic progression throughout the entire course of training. The object of such a progression is to achieve a peak of fitness from a relatively low starting point e.g. pre-season training, to intensive training which builds up speed, stamina and strength so that all are at a key pitch for the first competitive match.

Problems arise in football because this peak of fitness is required to last for nine months, and sometimes longer. This is virtually an impossibility! In comparison with the requirements of athletes, swimmers and boxers, who are able to gear their training to a relatively short session or to specific events so that they reach their physical peak at the appropriate time, the footballer is unable to descend from his physical peak, lose his sharpness and efficiency and re-charge his batteries ready for the build-up to the next peak. Thus, the whole process is more complex and intense for footballers and needs an examination of the training cycle (a term which illustrates the on-going nature of build-up, peak, recession which every athlete undergoes) at three distinct levels:

the programme for a full season;

that for a week;

that for each particular day.

From this it may appear that footballers do train harder, or at least ought to, than athletes and those participating in the other sports mentioned. There are many complicating factors which can affect any basic training programme for soccer – i.e. the number of games played within a certain period, type of opposition, position in table, current form, injuries, etc. Nevertheless, despite these extenuating factors, there are still clubs in both professional and amateur soccer (at top level and at village green level) who do not train their players objectively enough. What is much more relevant is that they do not train their players seriously enough, devising basic programmes of work related to the physical and psychological needs of the player, which can be adapted and manipulated as different conditions may dictate.

The intention of this chapter is to examine different facets of training, each having its own contribution towards the final product – namely to produce a player who is physically fit and alert to carry out efficiently the tasks asked of him in a game of football. As has been pointed out already, the key is *progression*. Bear this concept in mind and design a three-fold framework upon which to build (i.e. the season's, weekly and daily programme) for training sessions. Then the task of choosing one of the many activities which have accumulated over the years is simplified. Football training (and coaching) must have basic principles to clarify the many technical aspects (which are so often confusing).

Players are often required to participate in training sessions which are poor and pale imitations of something that their trainer has seen someone else put on, and even lead to players undergoing the wrong type of training.

It is not good enough merely to pay lip service to football training by presenting an ill-assorted mixture of activities which have been acquired over the years. Carefully compiled and well presented training schedules will not only produce a better pay-off physically but just as important, they will make each training session more meaningful to the player which in turn should produce a greater end product both in his physical condition and psychologically. The fact that the Club Trainer is dealing with a group of people who have to interact with each other makes the need for understanding the training requirements of footballers essential.

A systematic warming-up period before each training session will set the right pattern and create the right atmosphere for the activity to follow. The warm-up itself can be completed in a couple of minutes, or can take ten minutes or more, depending upon the future activity and its intensity.

Whether brief or extensive, the *warming-up period* should consist of comfortable free-running and stretching.

Phase I

Probably the easiest activity to organise which incorporates both ingredients is to have the players running around the the perimeter of the gym or training area in pairs, one pair behind the other. This enables the players to perform different types of running and exercises and yet remain organised. Exercises can be worked as the players jog around, including:
extending the arms sideways and returning;

high toe-raising;

kicking the heels up, behind;

toe-touching at a brisk walk;

jumping to head an imaginary ball;

and skipping and bringing the arms up high above the head, alternatively.

These and similar types of exercises supplement the various running activities, e.g.:

The last pair overtakes the others at a good stretch and become leaders;

last pair weave in and out of players in front of them;

backwards running;

sideways running with legs crossing;

sideways running with feet coming together and then apart;

changes of pace and direction with the emphasis on stretching the legs.

Phase II

If a more concentrated warm-up is required then the foregoing should be followed by a programme of continuous and more specific series of exercises and intensive sessions of running. These exercises, apart from their physical function of warming and stretching the muscles which are to be used violently in a short time, help to rivet the players' minds to the task in hand and can really set the adrenalin flowing, so giving a performance of higher quality. The exercises begin with the neck and work right through the body down to the ankles. Each exercise lasts between 10–20 seconds or 6–10 repetitions, and commences with the body relaxed from the exercises detailed in in Phase I. Phase II gradually increases in vigour, until by the time Phase III arrives the players are beginning to feel quite warm.

1. Neck rolling both ways, then stretching sideways to touch the shoulder with the ear, then backwards and forwards with chin on to the chest.

2. Arms and shoulders, front crawl, backstroke, breast stroke, butterfly both forwards and backwards.

3. Trunk bending sideways, legs straight, arm reaching as far down the legs as possible.

4. Hips circling both ways then forwards and back.

5. Stretching groins, legs wide apart and pushing body weight on to one leg and then on to the other.

6. Legs wide apart and straight, arms folded trying to touch the ground in front with the elbows.

7. Stretching hamstrings, legs together and kept straight with the feet crossed, pushing down with hands to touch the floor. Right foot over the left, and vice-versa.

8. Legs together, hands on knees and knees circling. Then push the knees forward and back.

9. Calf stretching, legs apart one in front of the other, increase the distance between them and put weight on the front leg until the calf of the rear leg pulls. Both heels must be on the floor during this exercise.

10. Ankle rotation both ways and forward and back.

11. Skip jumping and astride jumping mixed. Arms can be swung out and in, forward and backwards, with several high jumps, including spot runnings.

12. Five second sprint on the spot with everything (arms, legs, head) going.

It is important that there are no breaks between each exercise, so that the players are working continuously and their activity increases in intensity.

Phase III
The players then break into free running to round off the warming-up session by which time they are in top gear.
1. Running freely, trying to slap others on back or legs.
2. On command, chasing and slapping a named person. Change person often.

3. On command touching various parts of the gym or training area – again done quickly, so that the players are sprinting or moving quickly all of the time and are having to make rapid decisions.

The players are now ready to go straight into their training so maintaining the quality of work which has been progressively accumulated during the warm-up period.

Weight Training

The use of *weight training* has become very popular during the last two decades, and much time and effort is given to struggling under heavy loads that strain the back and ligaments of the limbs. The secret of weight training is to assess individual performance, because there is a wide variation between each player, and to allow him to train with weights that are comfortable and can be used repeatedly. For repetition is the key to successful weight training. It is not possible to generalise about this subject, but one of the most popular methods is the pyramid system where progression is achieved by increasing poundage while repetitions decrease – e.g. 10 repetitions at 50 lb. increasing by 10 lb. to 2 at 150 lb., and then up by 10 lb. to 200 or (x 2). But the diligent trainer must look out for the warning aches in the back, shoulders and knees. There is, of course, a real danger of damage to muscles and joints in weight training. The maximum lift for each player is recorded.

Stamina Training

Training also involves the gradual build up of stamina and speed. Once again it is difficult to specify certain techniques which are basically determined by the degree of fitness and ability of the players themselves. However, the key to *stamina training* is towards more extended use of interval training, when an oxygen debt is built up and a short rest period follows to allow recovery. This type of intermittent fast and slow exercise is more beneficial in increasing fitness than a moderate endurance run, but the physiological reasons for this fact are not known.

Basically, circuit training is just another method of stamina training, except that it is performed in a limited space with more variety of apparatus. By careful selection of the activities or exercises in the circuit the training can cater for strength, speed, muscular endurance and cardio-respiratory endurance. The minimum time for the circuit should be known (usually there are about 10 exercises) and the exercises can be maintained up to 30 minutes.

It is important to recall that a soccer player is called upon to perform a varied range of physical tasks over a period of 90 minutes. However, if a player lacks stamina he tires, and thus he performs the physical tasks less well as the game progresses – i.e. he runs more slowly, not as far or as often, he does not jump so high, and he takes longer to pick himself up when knocked over. The time he requires after performing a certain manoeuvre takes longer, and in general the physical challenge he imposes during a game diminishes, often rapidly. A footballer, however, is called upon to perform technical as well as physical tasks, and it is this part of his duties which suffers most when the player tires. At this period his oxygen debt increases and the muscles demand more oxygen, but the heart and lungs are unable to supply it. This in turn causes the players' selection processes to be impaired and mistakes follow. Overall, the player lacking stamina is unable to meet the physical and mental demands.

Before setting out the schedule for stamina development it is necessary to examine the type of running which takes place during a game of football. Apart from walking, jogging, running backwards and sideways and jumping, the average footballer during a game runs approximately 2,000 yards at a sprint at distances varying between 5 yards and 20 yards, and approximately 3,000 yards between half and full pace at varying distances up to 70 yards. These are very much approximate figures, but they give a very useful indication of the type of work required to build up the necessary stamina for such a performance. Also footballers do not always run in a straight line, but are required to stop and start, and change direction.

Thus shuttle running becomes the basis for stamina running. Once again it is convenient to divide the schedule into three parts.

Phase I

150-yard shuttles – e.g. start ... 5 yds ... 10 yds ... 15 yds ... 20 yds ... 25 yds. From the start each line is touched in turn, with the runner returning to touch the starting line; 150 yards are covered in this way. The time required is 35 seconds. It takes 14 similar shuttles to make up the 2,000 yards, and they are spread amongst other activities. However, many players would never tolerate such repetitions and other exercises are used.

The straightforward shuttle is easily organised with players going in relays e.g. 16 players in 4 groups, so that each group has 75 seconds rest between each shuttle. The selection side can be tested by having the distance markers in various directions from the middle so that the runner is aware of the next marker e.g.

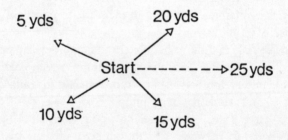

Running to different coloured bays or having to take out and bring back different coloured objects in a particular sequence makes the players think of selection, while obstacles add another dimension – e.g. poles to dodge around (body swerves), hurdles (jumping for the ball), and hurdles or benches to crawl under (quick recovery from falling during a match). When such obstacles are introduced then more time must be allowed.

Phase II

300-yard running. Up to 10 repetitions can be carried out – e.g. a straight 300 yards, or 6×50 yards with this distance being the minimum shuttle length. Time allowed for the straight 300 yards is 40 seconds. A variation can be running the length of a football pitch around the far goal posts and back; while team running also serves the same function – i.e. teams A and B line up at the half way line on the opposite sides of the pitch. Team A runs around the pitch where team B waits (approx. 200 yards, 30–35 seconds) and then jogs back across the centre line while team B sprints around to where team A originally stood.

In another variation the running load is gradually increased. Players start at the corner of a field, sprint to the centre line and jog the rest of the way to the start. They then sprint the length of the pitch and jog back, and so on, encompassing all corners of the field.

Phase III

This is a session which can be devised for inside or outside, and can be adapted to suit the required work load. This '100 per cent' session is basically the same as a circuit where a player must complete a given task in a certain time limit. The percentage aspect can be relaxed by demanding fewer repetitions of a task in the recognised 100 per cent time limit, or by allowing more time for the tasks.

	distance yds.	time secs.	between activity rest secs.	total time min. secs.
1. Across width of pitch and back (× 2).	280	20 each	35	1.50
2. 2 × 150 yard shuttles.	300	35 each	35	2.50
3. Physical contact activity.	—	—	—	2.00
4. Across goal area and back (× 3).	120	6 each	10	0.48
5. Half pitch shuttles (× 2).	300/316	35 each	35	2.20
6. Game.	—	—	—	2.00
7. 2 × 150 yard shuttles.	300	35 each	35	2.50
8. Across pitch and back plus 6 forward rolls.	140	30	30	1.00
9. Game (dodge and touch).	—	—	—	2.00
10. 2 × 150 yard shuttles.	300	35 each	35	2.50
	1,740			20.28

This is an example, but other activities can be included in the session but it is chiefly a running schedule and can be designed to total any given distance – e.g. 2,000, 3,000 or 4,000 yards.

Speed Training

Although there is some evidence to show that sprinters are born not made, there are a few steps by which some speed improvement can be achieved. These include an improvement of the basic mechanics or style of running, increasing strength/weight ratio including a reduction of body fat, adopting a correct stride length, and pre-tensing and co-ordinating the muscles before movement. So called 'power training' is commonly advocated to improve speed, with resistance to running applied by pressure from a partner or a machine (e.g. belt and treadmill).

Speed training is explosive work designed to improve performance in moving from a state of body inertia to full speed in as short a time as possible. Physical development to improve sprinting power is dealt with under weight training.

1. 90-yard shuttle where players go out 5 yards and back, repeating with 5-yard increments (e.g. 10, 15, 20 yards, etc.). These are short distances and require a quick turning and checking.

2. 10-yard and up to 25-yard dashes with inertia starts, such as facing the other way, squatting or hopping on haunches to the start line.

3. 20-yard races in pairs, one facing forwards, the other backwards (this player has 5 yards start).

4. Four 60-yard dashes, maximum time 8 seconds.

Again it must be emphasised that in many of these activities, especially shuttles, problems can be given to the players by arranging selections with coloured markers or shouted instructions.

5. Place changing, 10–15 yards or across the width of the gym, with players divided into teams of three or four. Each team is then subdivided so that one or two face across the course. All players are seated. One player from each team sprints across the gym and changes places with another opposite, who dashes across to where No. 1 came from, and so on. Players must sit until their turn for a run is due. This activity can be performed for 1-minute periods.

Chapter Nine

The Final Whistle

There are economic pressures on professional football clubs to devise quick and effective methods of treating injuries, since even the smallest injury can strike the club a severe financial blow. Exacting standards are required in football to ensure that the player recovers from his injury as quickly as possible. But there are no short cuts in treatment. This chapter examines several aids to recovery after injury which are commonly, and often uncritically, used.

One of the commonest abuses in the sporting scene is the use of a *local anaesthetic* injection to numb the injured area and allow a rapid return to the game. It has been reported that Stanley Matthews had a pain-killing injection before the 1953 Final; Pelé in 1966 and Beckenbauer in 1970 (*Sunday Times* 6th January, 1974). There is no doubt that there are exceptional circumstances when such an injection can be used (e.g. in a key, determined player before an important match which he or the team cannot afford to lose). But one should not forget that Perry, playing number 8 for the England rugby side in France, had six or eight injections into a damaged knee and played on. The fact that he had a comminuted fracture was missed, and the knee was so badly injured that he never played again.

Most club doctors are unhappy about giving a pain-killing injection, unless the injury is very superficial, e.g. a painful skin sore in a goalkeepers hand, a bruised small toe, minor teno-synovitis of wrist or ankle. Such injections must never be used in muscles, joints and ligaments. It is not unknown that after a pain-killing injection the injured tendon or muscle has completely torn, as in the case of Dorothy Tyler in the 1952 Olympics. Mary Rand also tore a tendon after being advised to have an injection.

Although the use of local anaesthetic injections is a subject of controversy, there is little argument in medical circles regarding the use of *plaster of Paris*. However, the need for a plaster must be clearly defined before one is used. Fractures in long bones (if not subjected to compression plating) require a plaster, as do severe ligament tears, joint effusions, recurrent synovitis of tendons and infections in limbs (e.g. cellulitis). It is noteworthy that in two seasons at Oxford only four plasters were used, two for cellulitis, and two to allow training after a fracture and a dislocation.

Thus the *advantages* of a plaster are:

rigid immobilisation;

relief of pain.

The *disadvantages* of a plaster are:

prolonged immobilisation of the injured area if allowed to remain for too long an interval depending upon the whim of the therapist or doctor, be he a 3-,5-,7- or 10-day man;

prevention of regular inspection of the injured area unless the plaster is split or applied as a backslab. Since the condition of sporting injuries can vary rapidly from day to day, this feature is an important consideration against the regular use of plaster;

causing muscle atrophy;

joint and cartilage degeneration, which may occur when a joint is kept fixed for over 3 weeks;

compression may be inadequate, it may be too tight initially and too slack as the swelling subsides;

dependent oedema may be found when the plaster is removed;

ulceration of the skin may be occasionally found;

the player walks with a poor movement pattern with leg plasters, usually the limb is rotated externally.

No one wishes to denigrate the time-honoured position of the plaster, but think before using one, and keep the duration of use to a minimum to avoid complications.

As has been previously mentioned, a firm *crêpe and wool bandage* (in several layers) gives comfortable and firm support especially in injuries around the knee. A U-adhesive *strapping* is excellent for ankle support, but adhesive should never be applied directly to the skin as it causes a great deal of pain on removal. Trainers must learn to apply a fine undercoat of tubi-grip or cotton bandage. Strapping can also be employed for finger injuries, wrist and shoulder sprains, toe and foot strains, and for minor fractures (e.g. fibular shaft). Often strapping can be used after a plaster has been removed – in the healing phase of a fracture – to prevent oedema and give some support. Mike Kearns, the Irish international goalkeeper, was treated by compression fixation after breaking his ankle, and for the next 7 days concentrated on remedial exercises as passive and gentle static exercises to the lower limb (as well as the more general body work). After 8 days he was mobile, non-weight-bearing on crutches, with a crêpe and wool support to prevent oedema and aid healing by guarding against excessive mobility. After 14 days a weight-bearing below-knee plaster was applied and the player began strenuous body work in the gym with the rest of the players. At this point he had a full range of movement in the injured ankle. Three weeks later the plaster was removed, and gentle mobilisation of the ankle and soft-ball kicking was commenced. By 7 weeks he had played in the Reserves. This case illustrated the full use of all forms of support in the average severe football injury, and their integration into a remedial exercise regimen.

*　　*　　*

Building up Muscle Power

This fact may be otherwise expressed as: Supporting the injured area is only part of treating the footballer as a whole, the emphasis should also be on mobilisation and remedial exercises to build up the internal struts of the body – the muscles.

Muscle testing after injury must be thoroughly carried out, because to build up muscle power the muscle must have a full range of movement. Players often suffer from tight hamstrings due to undertraining or rarely a back condition which reflexly causes tightness. Toe-touching with a standing player and a bent back gives some indication of hamstring tightness, but a further assessment can be made by getting the footballer to sit on a couch, flexing one knee to the abdominal wall to flatten out the lumbar spine, and then to reach towards his remaining foot. In this way the lumbar spine cannot compensate for any shortening in the hamstrings. Similarly the quadriceps can be tested by asking the player to flex the knee fully (any tightness causes restricted flexion) and then to kneel on the table and attempt to touch the table with his head by bending backwards. This test gives a powerful and sustained stretch to the quadriceps. An inability to fully point the toe downwards causes weakness in driving the ball. A simple method used in the England team was to ask the players to attempt to sit on their heels, the difference between buttocks and heel giving an accurate assessment of the restricted movement at the ankle. The Achilles tendon can be tested by getting the player to squat with his foot flat on the ground and gradually tilt the body weight forwards. This manoeuvre causes an aching in the affected tendon if it is not fully healed.

Although steroid injections can be given by the club doctor into damaged tendons, ligaments, etc., to reduce inflammation and to speed healing, their use requires some caution since repeated steroid injections can cause damage to fibrous and cartilaginous components, leading to weakness and perhaps rupture of the tendon or ligament concerned.

Heat Treatment

In the whole field of physical medicine no technique is more abused than the use of heat, either in infra-red, *short-wave diathermy* or *ultrasound* (although the latter has other effects). What are the real effects of heat? The obvious one of burning must not be ignored. However, there are other changes induced in the tissues by heat, namely increased blood flow, increased white cell migration, cell damage and oedema. The increased blood flow will promote haematoma formation and excessive scarring, if S.W.D. is applied during the initial stages of injury. However, short-wave is useful in promoting the feeling of comfort in a healing limb by relieving pain and has been said to aid re-absorption of tissue fluid. Gentle massage may also be of some benefit at this stage, but on the whole too vigorous massage has the risk of bone formation in the tissues. Ultrasound is not the panacea for all athletic troubles, although it is useful in chronic conditions, such as pulled tendons or muscles, and in the localisation of ligament injury. However, although ultrasound has been said to stimulate fibrous tissue formation, most of the micro-massage effects are probably due to a heating effect in the tissues.

It is beyond the scope of this book on injuries to detail all the therapeutic dosages and times of both ultrasound and S.W.D. It is important to point out that these electrotherapy methods are only part of a regimen which has the emphasis on rest and graduated activity. All sports injuries are different because of the variation between players and extent of injury. Therefore each player needs regular and constant supervision, and deployment of ultrasound and S.W.D. must be carefully considered in every case.

If a lesson or theme has emerged from this book, it should be that all football injuries require a common sense approach. As we have stated on many occasions there are no short cuts in treatment and the care of the injured sportsman requires patience and understanding. If there is a hope that emerges from this book, it is that more people will become interested in participating in sports, free from the worry of injury, and that at the end of a playing career they will partake in the coaching and care of others.

Truly, the football scene is a changing scene, and the treatment of the football injury needs constant reappraisal.

Index

141

Index